CASE STUDIES FOR THE EMERGENCY RESPONDER: PSYCHOSOCIAL, ETHICAL, AND LEADERSHIP DIMENSIONS

CASE STUDIES FOR THE EMERGENCY RESPONDER: PSYCHOSOCIAL, ETHICAL, AND LEADERSHIP DIMENSIONS

S. Joseph Woodall

and

Jeffrey A. Thomas

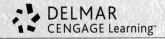

DELMAR
CENGAGE Learning

Australia • Brazil • Japan • Korea • Mexico • Singapore • Spain • United Kingdom • United States

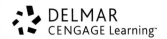

DELMAR
CENGAGE Learning™

Case Studies for the Emergency Responder: Psychosocial, Ethical, and Leadership Dimensions
S. Joseph Woodall and Jeffrey A. Thomas

Vice President, Career and Professional Editorial: Dave Garza

Director of Learning Solutions: Sandy Clark

Product Development Manager: Janet Maker

Managing Editor: Larry Main

Associate Product Manager: Meaghan O'Brien

Editorial Assistant: Amy Wetsel

Vice President, Career and Professional Marketing: Jennifer McAvey

Marketing Director: Deborah Yarnell

Senior Marketing Manager: Erin Coffin

Marketing Coordinator: Shanna Gibbs

Production Director: Wendy Troeger

Production Manager: Mark Bernard

Art Director: Benjamin Gleeksman

Library of Congress Control Number: 2 0 0 9 9 3 5 9 9 6

ISBN-13: 978-1-4180-5359-8

ISBN-10: 1-4180-5359-7

Delmar
5 Maxwell Drive
Clifton Park, NY 12065-2919
USA

Cengage Learning is a leading provider of customized learning solutions with office locations around the globe, including Singapore, the United Kingdom, Australia, Mexico, Brazil, and Japan. Locate your local office at: **international.cengage.com/region**

Cengage Learning products are represented in Canada by Nelson Education, Ltd.

To learn more about Delmar, visit **www.cengage.com/delmar**

Purchase any of our products at your local college store or at our preferred online store **www.CengageBrain.com**

Printed in the United States of America
1 2 3 4 5 6 7 13 12 11 10 09

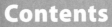
Contents

CASE STUDY 1
Knock-Knock

CASE STUDY 2
Rehab

CASE STUDY 3
A Penny for Your Thoughts

CASE STUDY 4
Fools Rush In

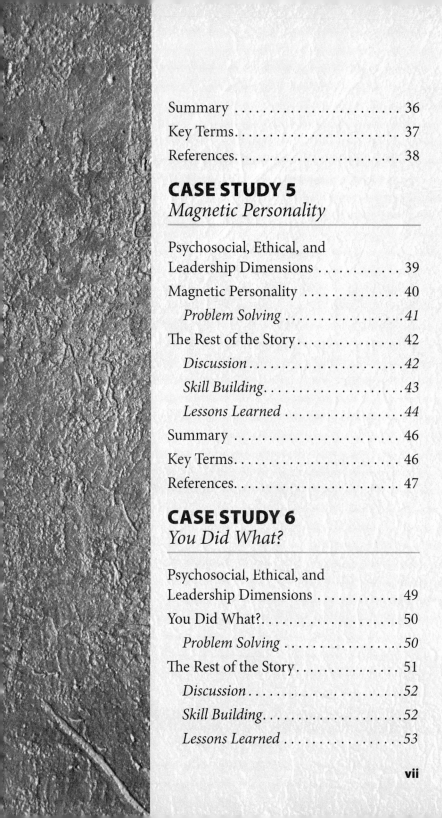

CASE STUDY 5
Magnetic Personality

CASE STUDY 6
You Did What?

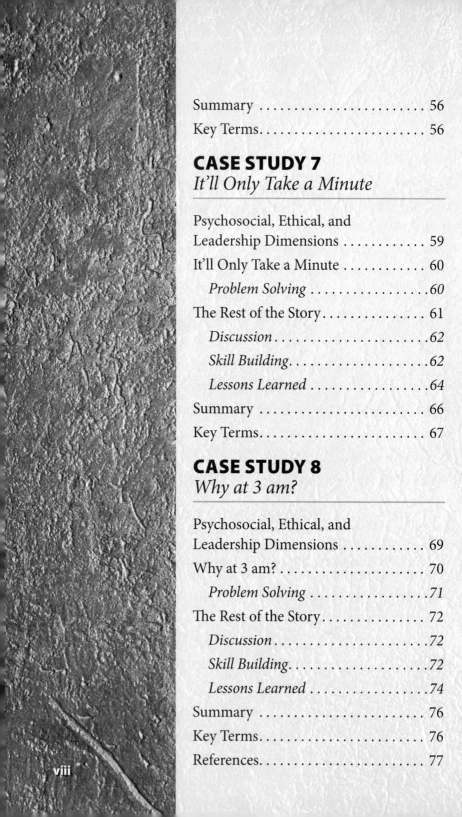

CASE STUDY 7
It'll Only Take a Minute

CASE STUDY 8
Why at 3 am?

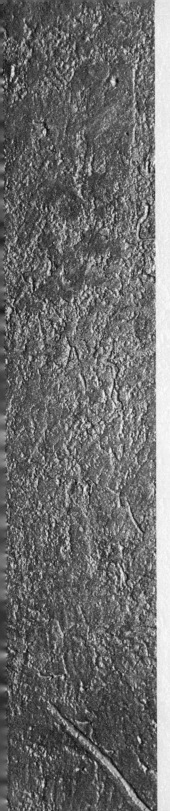

CASE STUDY 9
Where Do We Go from Here?

CASE STUDY 10
Bright Idea

CASE STUDY 13
Fatal Mistake

CASE STUDY 14
Holiday Get-Together

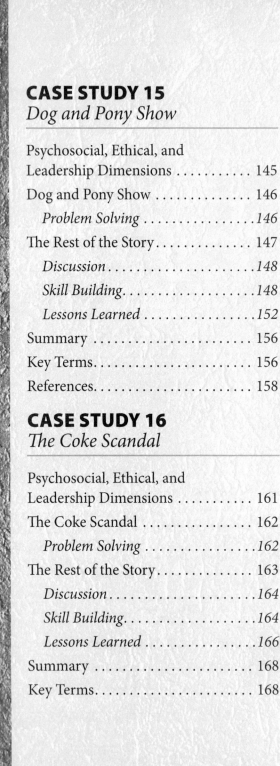

CASE STUDY 17
Crass Course

CASE STUDY 18
Cat on a Hot Tin Roof

CASE STUDY 19
All Dressed Up and No Place to Go

CASE STUDY 20
Food Poisoning

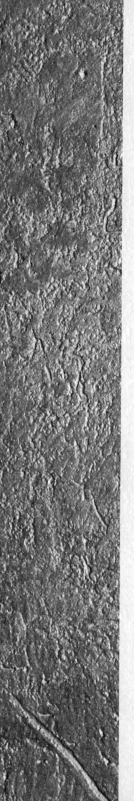

CASE STUDY 21
A Few Good Men

CASE STUDY 22
Appearances

CASE STUDY 23
A Quarter a Day
Keeps the Doctor Away

CASE STUDY 24
Professional Courtesy?

CASE STUDY 25
Frequent Flyer

CASE STUDY 26
This Is My Patient

CASE STUDY 27
The Perfect Storm

CASE STUDY 28
Family Ties

CASE STUDY 29
Salute

CASE STUDY 30
In Their Time of Grief

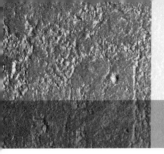

Preface

Emergency responders are frequently called upon to manage and mitigate incidents that are tragic. These types of calls challenge the very souls of these brave and caring men and women. Responders are also, though many times unwittingly, social workers, mediators, problem solvers, counselors, and sometimes simply someone willing to lend a hand. Consistently witnessing the tragedy and trauma of others can take an emotional toll leading to unhealthy and unsatisfactory coping mechanisms. Emergency response agencies are also charged with many other types of calls. These types of calls for service often seem to counter our mission and create stress. This stress may lead to what is characterized as compassion fatigue or burnout. These types of calls can bring out the best, and sometimes the worst, in a responder. They challenge our peoples' skills, initiative, attitude, innovation, and professionalism. How these challenges are framed and the actions that are subsequently taken are often career-defining events that are entered into an agency's oral history. *Case Studies for the Emergency Responder: Psychosocial, Ethical, and Leadership Dimensions* is dedicated to those who, no matter what the call, are obligated to respond and give each and every challenge their very best.

Concept

The case studies in this book have been designed to demonstrate how the interpersonal challenges of both the server and the served can be met head-on and effectively conquered. To accomplish this, we felt that it was necessary to provide cases of exemplary service and those that demonstrated social and professional clumsiness. We have intentionally sought a balance, firmly believing that there is as much to be learned from a positive example as from a negative one. We have also provided case studies spanning various psychosocial, ethical, and leadership topics.

These are not case studies breaking down any identifiable technical skill. Rather, they are examples of how different people react differently to a given set of rapidly changing and evolving circumstances. The strategies that are utilized by the responders demonstrate what can go right—actions leading to satisfactory outcomes, and what can go wrong—actions leading to a less than desirable outcome.

It is our goal for the reader to learn from the good examples, the clever, innovative, and professional interactions with patients, team members, and other public safety agencies. And to also learn from the poor examples that are often shortsighted, mundane, and unprofessional. We are hoping that these case studies will allow the veteran to reflect and the novice to grow, leading to meaningful discussions and dialogue in a variety of environments.

These case studies are all based on actual incidents and events. We have modified some case studies to improve readability and clarity, and to remove any identifiable information such as place, agency, and individual. Any similarities to agencies, individuals, or locations are coincidental and not intentional.

Organization

Each case study is broken down into nine sections. The first section identifies the specific psychosocial, ethical, and/or leadership dimensions that each story pertains to. The second section tells the story of a particular incident. Each incident is described to a point where it is evident that the responders are going to have to make a critical decision. The narrative stops and readers are presented with a section on problem solving, which provides a decision-making algorithm assisting the responder in evaluating the situation and making appropriate decisions. The algorithm is the same in each instance. The responder is asked to summarize what he or she knows about the situation and determine whether any further information or resources would be helpful to the decision-making process. The next step is an examination of the legal, ethical, organizational, or interpersonal responsibilities that come into play at this point in the scenario. Based on this analysis, the responder is asked to formulate an action plan. Once an action plan has been determined, the next step is to justify the plan and explain why this decision was made. The final step is to determine whether the plan requires any sort of follow-up.

After working through the decision-making algorithm, the reader is presented with the "The Rest of the Story" section. This section describes what steps were actually taken with regard to the incident. Sometimes these actions result in favorable outcomes and sometimes they do not. After reading this section, a list of discussion questions is presented. These questions allow the responder to critically evaluate what took place. They will also provide the opportunity to discuss alternative strategies. Instructors may find the questions useful for initiating classroom discussions. Following the "Discussion" section, the reader is presented with the "Skill Building" section. This section takes an in-depth look at the learning opportunities that are presented in each of the case studies. Some possible answers to each of the discussion questions can be found in this section. The next section takes a look at lessons learned. This section evaluates "The Rest of the Story" section using the decision-making algorithm. It is intended to show how the use of the algorithm may have prevented some negative outcomes. The "Summary" section of each case attempts to look at the bigger picture and the broader implications of the case presented. Key terms are listed to help both instructors and readers identify some of the more important points presented in each case.

Using This Book

This book has been designed so that it can be used in the classroom as a textbook, by agencies that are conducting initial training or providing continuing education, or for independent study. Each case is designed to be a stand-alone lesson. This allows for various applications. These cases can be used individually to supplement lessons by illustrating specific points that the instructor is trying to make. They can also be used as a supplemental text by having a class review of individual cases on a regularly scheduled basis. They can also be used as a stand-alone text. This book is equally well suited for use by emergency medical service (EMS) agencies and EMS education programs as well as by fire departments and fire education programs.

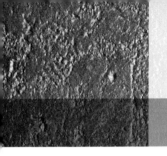

About the Authors

S. Joseph Woodall, Ph.D., NCC
Associate Professor and Director, Fire Science Program
Fayetteville State University
Fayetteville, NC

Dr. Joe Woodall is an Assistant Professor and the Director of the Fire Science Program at Fayetteville State University. His other university experience included three years as Visiting Assistant Professor in the Fire Safety Engineering Technology program at the University of North Carolina at Charlotte. Before this, he was the Division Chair and an Assistant Professor at Grand Canyon University in Phoenix, Arizona. While at Grand Canyon, he implemented and supervised the Public Safety Administration bachelor's degree program and the Master of Science in Executive Fire Service Leadership program.

Dr. Woodall holds a Ph.D. in Human and Organizational Systems and has a master's degree in Professional Counseling. He holds undergraduate degrees in Education and Fire Department Administration. He is also a graduate of the National Fire Academy's Executive Fire Officer Program.

Dr. Woodall retired from the City of Peoria, Arizona, Fire Department in July 2003. He actively served in all fire department ranks up to and including acting Battalion Chief but feels that his 12-year experience as a captain/emergency medical technician (EMT)/technical rescue technician on Ladder 193 made his contribution to this book meaningful.

Dr. Woodall has presented nationally on a variety of fire service topics and emergency responder mental health. He has worked as a therapist for the St. Luke's Behavioral Health Employee Assistance Program and is currently a Licensed Professional Counselor.

Jeffrey A. Thomas, Psy.D., NCC
Clinical Associate Professor
Arizona State University
City of Goodyear Fire Department
Goodyear, AZ

Dr. Jeff Thomas is a Clinical Associate Professor at Arizona State University. His primary responsibilities are teaching both graduate and undergraduate courses in fire service management. He conducts research in the area of fire and human behavior. He was recently named a senior fellow of the Lincoln Center for Applied Ethics and has focused on applied ethics for emergency responders.

Dr. Thomas received his Doctor of Psychology Degree from the University of Northern Colorado and practiced in Phoenix, Arizona, for a decade. He has extensive experience treating public safety professionals both in his private practice and while working for an employee assistance program. He has been a member of the Goodyear Fire Department for eight years and is currently assigned as Emergency Management Coordinator. While in college, he worked as an EMT for Life Ambulance in Wheat Ridge, Colorado.

Dr. Thomas has provided consultation to many fire departments and EMS agencies throughout the United States and Canada. He is recognized internationally as an expert in the areas of juvenile firesetting and adult arson. He has also been involved in paramedic education and training for many years. He offers classes to paramedics and others to help them improve their ability to respond to psychological emergencies and provide a higher-level of customer service.

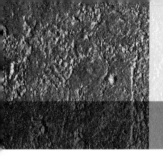

Acknowledgments

The authors gratefully acknowledge the following individuals, agencies, and institutions for their assistance and support during the writing of these case studies:

Jodi Woodall
Alexis Woodall
Lindsay Woodall
Drake Woodall
Andrew McCarthy
Captain Patrick Doyle, CEP
Captain Wade Denny, CEP
City of Goodyear, Arizona, Fire Department
City of Fayetteville, North Carolina, Fire Department
City of Albemarle, North Carolina, Fire Department
The crews of Fayetteville Fire Department-Station 14
The firefighters of the City of Peoria, Arizona, Fire Department
Fayetteville State University
Arizona State University
Delmar Cengage Learning

The authors would also like to thank the reviewers for their valuable feedback and expertise.

Questions and Feedback

The authors are interested in hearing your stories as well. We encourage our readers to submit any of their stories that they feel would be helpful to others. Please send your stories to us at:

S. Joseph Woodall, Ph.D.: jwoodall@uncfsu.edu
Jeffrey A. Thomas, Psy.D.: jeffrey.a.thomas@asu.edu

Delmar Cengage Learning also welcomes your questions and feedback. To send us your questions or feedback, you can contact the publisher at:

Delmar Cengage Learning
Executive Woods
5 Maxwell Drive
Clifton Park, NY 12065
Attn: Emergency Medical Services Team

We have enjoyed putting this collection together and hope you would enjoy reading and learning from these stories.

Sincerely,
S. Joseph Woodall, Ph.D.
Jeffrey A. Thomas, Psy.D.

Knock-Knock

Psychosocial, Ethical, and Leadership Dimensions

- Community Relations
- Customer Service
- Public–Private Partnerships
- Public Education

Knock-Knock

The four-person ALS Engine Company had just settled in their recliners to watch *Monday Night Football*. The meal was sitting heavy and they were ready to take a much deserved break. The dispatch lights came on and they heard the familiar, "Channel 9 Medical Alarm." The groans, complaints, and strain filled the dayroom. "C'mon," said the captain, "let's make this a quick one and get back for the second quarter."

The run was just a few blocks from the station and with little haste the engine pulled up at a well-manicured residence. The routine was well practiced, so the crew and the gear reached the front door in a rapid fashion. Their knocking and yelling received no response. "Well, this is great," stated the engineer/paramedic, "looks like we're going to have to break in."

The captain/EMT sent the firefighter back to the truck for the forcible entry tools while the remaining crew members started toying with the window screens. They selected the small kitchen window facing the street as the point for the forcible entry and were just about to break the window to gain entry.

Problem Solving

What Do You Know?

- Describe what you know about this incident.

What Do You Need to Know?

- What additional information is required before further decision making?

Resources

- What potential resources would be helpful at this stage?

Responsibilities

- What legal, ethical, organizational, or interpersonal responsibilities should you consider?

Action Plan

- Decide what you would do next if you were in this situation.

Justification of Your Action Plan

- Explain the rationale you used for your decision.

Follow-up

- Would your action plan require any follow-up? Why or why not?

The Rest of the Story

Just as they were about to break the window, they were interrupted by a feeble, squeaky voice. "Hello boys, what are you doing?" They collectively turned around to see an elderly woman walking up to their location.

They said, "Well ma'am, someone in this house pushed their medical alarm and now we can't get them to open the door. We're afraid that the person might be unconscious and dying so we're going to break in so that we can help them."

"Oh my, this is terrible," she chortled.

"Why? Do you know who lives here?" asked the firefighter/EMT.

"Why yes, yes I do," she replied with a distant smile.

"Well do you know if they've been sick or are disabled or hard of hearing," queried the engineer/paramedic.

"No, it's nothing like that. Actually, I live here," she self-consciously replied.

"Does anyone live here with you?" asked the firefighter/EMT.

"No, I live here all alone. Fred, my husband, died a couple of years ago. You see, I was over at Hazel's house and was wondering if this thing would work if I was away from home," she stated tugging on her new medical alarm necklace. "So I pushed the button and just watched from Hazel's kitchen window."

Seeing the humor in all this, the captain/EMT chose to make this incident a learning moment and politely explained the medical alert system. All parted in good spirits and with a good laugh. The woman returned to Hazel's kitchen and the engine company returned to the station for the second quarter of the football game.

Discussion

- Was the immediate situation handled correctly?
- Did the woman who activated the medical alarm do anything wrong?
- How might this call have had a negative outcome?
- What responsibility does the medical alarm company have in educating their customers?
- What could EMS agencies do to prevent this from occurring?

Skill Building

Responses such as this tax a service designed to assist the sick and injured. They also create a great deal of stress and consternation with responders. We can only reframe them as opportunities to demonstrate our customer service skills and as an opportunity to enhance public relations. As such, the captain of this crew made a good choice. Had he chosen to chastise this woman, he likely would have caused some hurt feelings and embarrassment. Furthermore, the woman may have some reluctance to use her medical alarm in an actual emergency. This woman meant no harm by her actions. She did not have the knowledge to fully understand how her actions impact the EMS system. She was merely trying to learn the limitations of her medical alert system.

Reframing the challenge, however, is not a long-term solution to a dilemma that will probably increase as our population continues to age. Measures that can be designed and implemented in an effort to reasonably and cost-effectively meet the needs of our citizens should be examined and undertaken. This case study also describes a public–private interaction. A medical alarm company provides their customers with a sense of security. This is a good thing but does not come without some responsibility on the part of the company. While they sell, install, repair, and monitor the system, it is, in most cases, a public service that responds to the alarm. The growing number of calls, such as the one described here, have identified the need for some much needed public education. Most fire and EMS agencies have public education programs. These field delivered programs provide education on fire safety behaviors, smoke alarms, cardiopulmonary resuscitation (CPR), first aid, fire extinguishers, home safety, and injury prevention, to name a few. It could be argued that the proper use of medical alarms should be added to the public education menu.

The introduction of any new product usually produces unintended consequences. This situation represents one of them. Although it defies logic, it happened and has most likely repeated itself throughout the country. This case study calls for public–private interagency cooperation in the area of public education. Because the medical alarm company is a for-profit business, they could furnish the hard copy educational material and the various public education programs that already exist could deliver the information.

Lessons Learned

What Do You Know?

This crew has been summoned to an unknown emergency through a private medical alarm monitoring agency. On arrival they were unable to make contact with the patient as they were locked out of the residence.

What Do You Need to Know?

Try before you pry is the standard procedure. Are there any other points of entry that would provide patient access? Crew members should check all doors and windows prior to initiating forcible entry. It would also be advisable to check with dispatch, making sure that the emergency responders are at the correct address. The pessimistic approach must drive the course of action in this scenario. It must be assumed that the person, or persons, in the residence are unresponsive, unable to unlock the door, or call out for help.

Resources

The emergency medical dispatcher could prove to be a valuable resource in this situation. The captain/EMT would want to contact dispatch and request a callback number to the residence. If the dispatch system has this information, a callback should be requested. The captain/EMT should also request dispatch to contact the medical alarm monitoring agency, checking whether any other method of contact, such as a cell phone, is available.

If the local law enforcement has not been notified, it is always good practice to request that they be dispatched. Time constraints may not allow the responding providers to wait for them to arrive. If forcible entry, in the judgment of the crew, must take place prior to the arrival of law enforcement, they should still be summoned. They will be able to document the necessity of forcible entry and assist in securing the residence after the situation has been mitigated.

Potential patient downtime is a critical factor. However, if enough personnel are present, it would be advisable to send crew members to the adjacent houses and even to the neighbors across the street to see if anyone has a key or additional information that may be of help, even while forcible entry is taking place.

Responsibilities

Ethically speaking, the responding agency has the responsibility to make patient contact by whatever means necessary. Again, it must be assumed that the patient, or patients, are unable to provide entry. Organizationally, operations orders and EMS protocols justify an action plan incorporating forcible entry. Interpersonally, the entire crew is responsible for building positive community relations and taking the high road when approaching their interaction in a positive, congenial manner.

Action Plan

The decision to force entry is a sound and defendable action plan. It must be assumed that the patient, or patients, are unresponsive and unable to assist in their own rescue until proven otherwise. In this case, contact with the patient was made before forcing entry. It was at this juncture that the action plan shifted from a rescue plan to a community relations opportunity.

Justification of Your Action Plan

Emergency responders must always err in the favor of the patient. When patients are unable to act in their own behalf, it is the EMS responders' responsibility to act for them. If acting in their favor requires the destruction of property, then such destruction is justified. If the responding crew expeditiously exhausted any and all avenues to establish patient contact—notifying dispatch, asking dispatch to contact the medical alarm monitoring agency, requesting law enforcement, and checking all points of entry prior to forcing entry—then their action plan would be fully justifiable.

Follow-up

Follow-up in this scenario would examine ways to prevent this from occurring in the future. The captain/EMT would be wise to contact the next higher level in the command structure to explain what happened on this call. This conversation could initiate an examination of the working relationship between the public EMS provider and the medical alarm monitoring agency. An examination of this public–private partnership may lead to a long range mitigation plan designed to educate the consumer on the proper manner in which to utilize the medical alarm service.

Summary

This case study offers lessons on several levels. At the interpersonal level, it exhibits how important it is for the emergency responder to "reframe" an encounter with the public as a community relations opportunity. By deciding to approach this situation as a learning opportunity, the captain/EMT placed the agency he represents, and himself, in a positive light. The action plan in this scenario also demonstrates sound and positive customer service. No feelings were hurt and no one left the encounter angry. The woman in this encounter made a mistake, most likely due to inadequate information about the medical alarm and the emergency agency's dispatch and response system.

This response also shed light on the importance of a comprehensive public education program. Had the medical alarm monitoring company fully educated the customer, this situation may have been entirely prevented. Because, evidently, the medical alarm monitoring company did not explain that the medical alert alarm was tied solely to the address of her residence and not to the location that the user was at, it was almost inevitable that a scenario such as this would occur. The long-term solution to prevent future occurrences such as this would most likely involve a public–private partnership or, if both agencies were private, a private–private partnership directed at fully and completely educating the consumer of the functions and limitations of the medical alarm system. The details and mechanics of just how such a partnership would work could be worked out on a case-by-case basis.

Finally, it is important for those working at the service delivery end of an agency's continuum to recognize, understand, and acknowledge that each call for service impacts the organization at many, many levels. It is through this recognition, understanding, and acknowledgment of these levels that the emergency responder can provide the best service possible with minimum consternation and angst.

Key Terms

Community Relations   The process of building political and public support within the organization, the emergency response system, with policy makers and with the community.

Public Education   Comprehensive wellness and injury prevention programs designed to eliminate or mitigate situations that risk the lives or health of the public.

Public–Private Partnership   Formal or informal interagency agreements designed to enhance a given system of service or a process in the interest of the end consumer.

Medical Alarm   An automated electronic notification device worn on, or kept near to, the subscriber. When activated, a signal is transmitted to a monitoring agency, which in turn notifies the appropriate emergency medical provider.

2

Rehab

Psychosocial, Ethical, and Leadership Dimensions

- Ethics
- Fitness for Duty
- Hostile Work Environment
- Supervision

Rehab

Jason was excited about his new job at Star Ambulance, a private company that served a small town neighboring the town where he had grown up. He had been going to night classes at the hospital for the past several months and had become a certified emergency medical technician. This job was the payoff and he was on top of the world. He felt like he had arrived.

Jason was assigned to the day shift on Ambulance 2. While he was on probation, he would be working with two older EMTs and learn how the company worked. Ricky and Steve had been working together for several years. Management trusted them to supervise and train all the new employees. Jason was a bright young man and an enthusiastic student. He was eager to develop all the skills he had learned.

Jason worked hard. He soon discovered that the bulk of Star Ambulance's business was inter-facility transports. They occasionally went on emergency calls when a county unit was not unavailable. Jason enjoyed the rush he felt when working at an emergency scene. He could not understand why his mentors preferred the slower pace of inter-facility transports.

After having worked there for a couple of months, Jason arrived for work one Sunday morning. He was surprised by what he found. Steve was standing out back behind the ambulance garage breathing from an oxygen mask. Ricky was just about to stick him with an IV needle. "Hi Jason, you're early this morning," Ricky said casually.

"What's wrong with Steve?" exclaimed Jason.

"I'm OK. I'll be fine in a few minutes," Steve mumbled through the mask.

"He just had a hard night of drinking. I'm going to fix him up with a little saline and he'll be good as new," explained Ricky.

Problem Solving

What Do You Know?

- Describe what you know about this incident.

What Do You Need to Know?

- What additional information would be helpful before further decision making?

Resources

- What potential resources would be helpful at this stage?

Responsibilities

- What legal, ethical, organizational, or interpersonal responsibilities should you consider?

Action Plan

- Decide what you would do next if you were in this situation.

Justification of Your Action Plan

- Explain the rationale you used for your decision.

Follow-up

- Would your action plan require any follow-up? Why or why not?

The Rest of the Story

Jason didn't know what to say. He just stood there with his mouth open. These were men he respected and trusted as EMS professionals. "What's the matter?" asked Steve. "Cat got your tongue?"

"Uh, no," stammered Jason.

"Look," said Ricky, "this is just one of those things that happen sometimes. You stay out a little bit too late, you have a little bit too much to drink; you're just not all there when it comes time to start your shift. You come to work, breathe oxygen for about fifteen minutes, take in a liter of saline, and wah-lah, your hangover is gone."

"This is just something we can do to help each other out," added Steve. "Someday it will be your turn." Jason didn't know what to say. He just stood there as Ricky started the IV in Steve's arm. Ricky and Steve made small talk as the IV bag drained. When the bag was empty, Ricky removed the IV and threw all of the equipment into the red biowaste container. The three of them went inside the quarters and Steve told the dispatchers that they were available for service.

They sat down together at the table in the break room. Steve and Ricky looked at Jason. "I know that you like working here," Steve said to Jason. "There are some things that happen in EMS that you just have to keep quiet about."

"This is one of those times," added Ricky.

"It is important that your partner be able to trust you," continued Steve. "I know that you are new, if you want to fit in around here you are going to have to learn when to keep your mouth shut. Sometimes you are going to see and hear things that you don't like. That is just part of working on an ambulance."

"We know that you want to make it through probation," Ricky affirmed. "Steve and I are going to remember this when we write your evaluation."

Discussion

- Do you think that Ricky and Steve's behavior was ethical?
- Did Ricky and Steve violate any policies and procedures?
- Did Ricky and Steve violate any laws?
- What should Jason have done in this situation?

Skill Building

There are several problematic factors here. The first is whether Steve is fit for duty. It appears that Steve did not report to work in a condition that would allow him to work. If he was truly in need of oxygen and IV fluids, it is clear that he was unfit for duty and could not adequately perform his duties as an EMT. Steve's duties likely include driving the ambulance, assessing and treating patients, starting IVs, and administering medications. We would hope that his agency has a policy regarding the condition an employee should be in when he or she reports to work. Steve places his agency and his professional certification in jeopardy by reporting to work in the condition he was in.

Ricky becomes complicit in the problem when he agrees to administer the IV to Steve. Although he may be able to adequately perform his duties, he now assumes the professional liability for Steve being able to perform his duties as well. He also shares in the responsibility for putting his agency at risk and has placed his professional certification at risk. In addition, both Ricky and Steve are guilty of theft from their employer and have likely violated polices relating to employee theft. No doubt the agency's administrators would take a dim view of this behavior.

Moreover, Steve and Ricky have also placed Jason in a very difficult position. He is a new employee who has now become witness to a number of policy violations, criminal behavior, and a breach of professional ethics. The situation is compounded by the fact that Steve and Ricky directed Jason to keep quiet if he wanted to continue working there and that he would be rewarded for his silence when the time comes for his evaluation. This behavior constitutes a hostile work environment. A hostile work environment exists when there is an offensive, intimidating, or oppressive environment (Varone, 2007). Ricky and Steve threatened Jason's continued employment based on his willingness to become an accomplice in their unprofessional behavior. If Jason does comply, he risks his entire professional future. If he does not comply, he faces the possibility of having to continue in a hostile work environment and the possibility of further threats and intimidation. He also allows this type of environment to continue and increases the possibility that other employees may be subjected to similar behavior.

If Jason reports the behavior, he runs the risk of being singled out and ostracized by his coworkers.

No EMS or fire service professional should be subjected to a hostile work environment. This type of behavior is dishonorable and is also illegal (Varone, 2007). Jason should follow the chain of command and report this situation to Steve and Ricky's supervisor. He should also take the time to document what he has seen. If Jason reports a hostile work environment, he is protected under the law (Varone, 2007). It is incumbent on the supervisor to take action. He or she should investigate the report and take the appropriate disciplinary action. If Steve and Ricky deny their behavior, the supervisor should take steps to reassign Jason and allow him to complete his probation on another ambulance and/ or shift.

Lessons Learned

What Do You Know?

Jason is a probationary employee who witnessed professional misconduct by his immediate supervisors. This misconduct includes a number of policy violations, possible criminal activity, and a breach of professional ethics. Furthermore, Jason is given direction to look the other way and not report this behavior if he wants to continue working for this agency. In addition to the policy violations, there are obvious safety issues. If Steve is not fit for duty, he could be placing both Jason and Ricky at risk if he drives the ambulance. There is also the increased risk that Steve may make a mistake when treating a patient. This puts the public at risk. Steve also risks his professional certification and the professional certification of his crew members in the event of something going wrong.

What Do You Need to Know?

What are Star Ambulance's policies regarding fitness for duty and the use of company property for personal gain? Furthermore, Jason should be aware of any statutes or professional regulations that apply. It is also important for Jason to understand the company's policy regarding a hostile work environment and what is the correct procedure for reporting one.

Resources

It would be wise to consult the agencies policy manual regarding the behavior that was witnessed and what is the organizational expectation of an employee who witnessed the behavior. If Jason is still unsure about what to do, he may want to consult someone outside the agency. He could speak to one of his instructors from the hospital or one of his former classmates. If this is not possible, he could always speak to someone whose judgment he trusted that is outside the EMS industry. This outside perspective is oftentimes very useful in working through ethical dilemmas. If Jason is consulting with other EMS professionals, he should take care to describe the situation in its general terms and not reveal the names of the other individuals.

Star Ambulance likely has a policy on hostile work environments and the procedure for employees who feel that they are being subjected to one. Jason should consult the policy manual or speak to Steve and Ricky's supervisor. The Internet is also a good resource for general information and federal laws that apply to hostile work environment.

Responsibilities

Jason has legal, ethical, and organizational responsibility to report this behavior. He also has the interpersonal responsibility to speak with Ricky and Steve about the behavior that he finds objectionable. EMS professionals share a responsibility in monitoring their own. No EMS professional should allow another to practice when they are not fit for duty. We all have an obligation to watch out for the safety of ourselves, each other, and the public.

Action Plan

The wise thing for Jason to have done would have been to document what had happened. The documentation should include the date and the time of the events; it should also include as many direct quotes as possible. Jason should then request a meeting with management and report what had happened. It may be wise to write a memo requesting a meeting and indicate that the subject is a hostile work environment. By putting this in writing, Jason would be protected from any type of retribution.

Justification of Your Action Plan

Jason must report what happened or he becomes complicit in all the policy violations and the illegal activity. If he chooses not to say anything, he places his entire future as an EMT at risk. If this story resulted in a driving accident or an error in patient care, an investigation would surely follow. It is highly likely that these events would be uncovered in the investigation.

If Jason chose to confront Ricky and Steve at the table in the break room, the result could have been disastrous. He was outnumbered by two to one and was already being threatened. The supervisors could have invented a story to cover-up their behavior or found some way to get back at Jason. By documenting the incident and submitting a memo to management, Jason protects himself, the ambulance company, and the public. This type of behavior has no place in EMS and should not be tolerated or condoned in any way.

Follow-up

Management needs to follow-up on the complaint. The complaint would likely initiate an internal investigation. Management may want to conduct supervisory training for all of the company's supervisors. Reporting the behavior also places Jason in a difficult position. He should document any further threats or mistreatment. He should also request a different supervisor for the rest of his probationary period and if possible avoid working with Ricky and Steve in the future.

Summary

This case illustrates that sometimes we can find ourselves in difficult situations through no actions of our own. Even though it may difficult, the best way out of these situations is to do the right thing.

An EMS professional will always survive these situations by taking a strong ethical stance and following organizational policies. Many of us develop close friendships with the people we work with. Some might say that a loyal friend would look the other way and keep quiet. This attitude can create an internal conflict between that loyalty and doing the right thing. It could be argued that any friend who puts another friend in this type of situation is taking advantage of that loyalty. Don't make the mistake of confusing friendliness with true friendship.

This case is made more complex by the fact that Ricky and Steve were not Jason's friends; they were his supervisors. Supervisors have a responsibility to see that all employees are treated fairly and equally. In addition to all of the violations and illegalities, Ricky and Steve were certainly not being fair to Jason. Creating a hostile work environment is an example of supervision at its worst. Federal and state laws exist to protect employees in any industry from being forced to work in a hostile environment. Hopefully, the management of this company would not allow this type of behavior to continue.

As EMS professionals, we all have the obligation to arrive at work in a condition that will allow us to perform at the highest level. The public expects us and trusts us to be at our best when we arrive at an emergency scene. To arrive at work in condition that makes us unfit for duty is an egregious violation of the public's trust.

Key Terms

Ethics   The ability to make sound decisions based on what is considered right and wrong, what is morale, and what is legal.

Fitness for Duty   The physical and mental health status of an employee that allows for the performance of essential job duties in an effective and safe manner and protects the health and safety of oneself, coworkers, and the public.

Hostile Work Environment   A hostile work environment exists when there is an offensive, intimidating, or oppressive environment.

Supervision   The action carried out to oversee the productivity and progress of employees who report directly to an individual.

References

Varone, C. J. (2007). *Legal Considerations for Fire and Emergency Services.* Clifton Park, NY: Thomson-Delmar Learning.

3

A Penny for Your Thoughts

Psychosocial, Ethical, and Leadership Dimensions

- Child Abuse
- Cultural Differences

A Penny for Your Thoughts

Squad 51 had just changed shifts. John and Roy were busy checking out all their equipment when the first call came over the loudspeaker. "Squad 51. Ill child. 1444 South Palm Lane. Time out 0712." John picked up the radio, "Squad 51 responding. KMG 365." They left the station and responded Code 3 to the address in a part of town known as Little Vietnam.

Upon arrival, they were shown to a bedroom where a 7-year-old girl was lying in bed. The family was present, but the parents did not speak much English. John and Roy began their assessment. Fortunately, the girl spoke better English than her parents. Their assessment revealed that the little girl was somewhat listless and tachycardic. Her blood pressure was slightly elevated, her breathing was labored, and she had a temperature of 102°F. When John sat her up to listen to her lungs, he discovered that the back of her neck was covered with red welts.

"Roy, take a look at this," John said with a strong look of concern on his face.

Roy leaned over to look at the girl's neck. "Yeah" was all he said as he nodded at his partner in silent agreement.

John proceeded to listen to the girl's lungs and determined that there was some bilateral wheezing. He also did a complete head to toe examination and found no other signs of welts or bruising.

Problem Solving

What Do You Know?

- Describe what you know about this incident.

What Do You Need to Know?

- What additional information would be helpful before further decision making?

Resources

- What potential resources would be helpful at this stage?

Responsibilities

- What legal, ethical, organizational, or interpersonal responsibilities should you consider?

Action Plan

- Decide what you would do next if you were in this situation.

Justification of Your Action Plan

- Explain the rationale you used for your decision.

Follow-up

- Would your action require any follow-up? Why or why not?

The Rest of the Story

Roy patched with Rampart General and reported the findings. They were instructed to give the girl some oxygen and transport her as soon as possible. Roy did his best to explain that they would be taking the girl to Rampart, that the mother could ride in the ambulance with her, and that the rest of the family would have to follow by automobile. Following the ambulance to the hospital, John and Roy discussed the welts on the back of her neck. They both agreed that they would need to report their suspicions of child abuse.

In the emergency room, they gave their report to Dr. Morten and voiced their concerns about suspected child abuse. Dr. Morten examined the girl and concluded that she was suffering from pneumonia. When he asked the girl what happened to her neck, she explained that her grandmother had been rubbing the back of her neck with the edge of a penny several times a day for the past three days. Dr. Morten asked Nurse McCall to contact the hospital social worker.

Discussion

- Do you think John and Roy were correct to suspect child abuse?
- Was it wrong for them not to ask any questions about the welts on the girl's neck?
- What was their responsibility for reporting suspected child abuse?
- How will you handle the reporting of suspected child abuse?
- In your jurisdiction, to what agency do you report suspected child abuse?

Skill Building

EMS providers are mandatory reporters of child abuse in every jurisdiction. Failure to report suspected abuse is a violation of standard EMS protocols and state statutes. A good report of child abuse must include a description of the patient, his or her chief complaint, medical findings, medications and compliance, any known diagnoses, his or her mental status, lethality assessment, and a brief psychosocial history (Thomas & Woodall, 2006). The assessment of abusive situations must be reported to the local child protective services and/or local law enforcement according to protocols and state laws. EMS responders may also be able to report suspected abuse to the receiving hospital. Hospitals frequently have social workers or other mental health professionals who handle child abuse reports. No matter what the reporting mechanism, it is important for EMS providers to document suspected abuse and to whom they reported it. It is not the responsibility of the EMS provider to determine whether child abuse actually occurred; that is the responsibility of other professionals. Our responsibility is simply to report any and all suspected abuse.

    John and Roy were correct to suspect abuse in this situation. The welts on the girl's neck could have been caused by any number of things such as allergic reactions, insect bites, or other medical conditions. They could also be the result of physical abuse, strangulation, or restraint. They might also have been caused by some type of home remedy such as hot towels or massage.

In this case, the welts on the girl's neck were the result of a traditional form of healing practiced by many Asian cultures. The treatment, known as coin rubbing, involves rubbing the body forcefully with a coin. This rubbing almost always produces red welts. In some cases, the coin may be heated with a candle or coated with a balm before the rubbing. Many reports of successful healing through this practice have been reported (Davis, 2000).

Many cultures practice forms of healing that are very different from conventional western medicine. Typically, we are only contacted when the traditional healing methods have failed. It is important to assess the healing methods of different cultures in your community so that these practices do not distract from doing a thorough patient assessment. In this case, the young girl was not a victim of child abuse. In fact, the grandmother's coin rubbing was a caring act of love and nurturance.

Lessons Learned

What Do You Know?

Squad 51 responded to an ill child call in a predominately ethnic neighborhood. John and Roy assessed and treated a 7-year-old Asian girl. Their assessment showed listlessness, tachycardia, slight hypertension, labored breathing, and a temperature of 102°F. They also observed red welts on the back of the girl's neck. She was transported to the hospital where she was diagnosed and treated for pneumonia. When asked about the welts on her neck, the girl explained that for the past few days her grandmother had been rubbing the back of her neck with a penny. The treating physician requested the hospital social worker to assess for possible child abuse.

What Do You Need to Know?

EMS providers should be familiar with the signs and symptoms of abuse. Although it is not our role to investigate abuse, we must be familiar enough with the signs and symptoms to be in a position to assess and report suspected abuse. Providers must be familiar with their agency's procedures for reporting abuse.

Resources

Most EMS systems have a resource for consultation on suspected abuse. This may be a hospital social worker or other mental health provider. EMS providers can always call a supervisor for consultation or request that a supervisor report to the scene. In some cases, it may also be prudent to request that law enforcement respond to the scene.

Responsibilities

EMS providers are legally mandated to report suspected abuse. Failure to do so is a violation of the law and a breach of professional protocols.

Action Plan

The proper plan in this case is to follow your agency's procedures for reporting abuse. Be sure to document all of your findings and to whom the report was made. If possible, make sure that you are given a case number and include it in your documentation.

Justification of Your Action Plan

EMS providers are legally mandated to report suspected abuse.

Follow-up

It is recommended that a supervisor be notified that suspected abuse has been reported. This allows for the agency to be prepared in the event of a criminal or civil trial. Reporting child abuse can be a stressful and emotional activity for an EMS provider. Notifying a supervisor also allows the supervisor to assess for a stress reaction and provide a debriefing or other form of critical incident stress management if one is indicated. This agency may want to consider some training or an educational memo regarding coin rubbing be provided to their employees.

Summary

This case is a good example of how cultural differences can affect the outcome of call. A vast number of traditional or different healing practices exist in the community. It would be impossible to be familiar with them all. However, it may be wise to examine the healing practices of different cultures that are represented in your community. This awareness may help us from reaching a conclusion without having all the available facts.

No EMS provider wants to encounter cases of child abuse. Unfortunately, it is not possible to get through a career in this field without encountering this tragedy. In 2005, an estimated 3.3 million referrals, involving the alleged maltreatment of approximately 6 million children, were made to child protective service agencies in the United States (Hopper, 2007). Make sure that you take good care of yourself and your crewmates after you encounter one of these situations. Make sure to talk through the incident and identify any thoughts and feelings that you are experiencing. It is also advisable to exercise within 24 hours of a difficult call.

Key Terms

Child Abuse Report   Child abuse and neglect is the subject of mandatory reporting for EMS providers in all jurisdictions.

Coin Rubbing   A legitimate treatment practice in traditional Chinese medicine that is practiced just as much by highly trained experts as it is practiced by the folk users. It should be viewed as an immediate form of domestic first-aid intervention that serves to prevent any need for further medical treatment.

Cultural Differences   This term reflects the differences among the people that EMS agencies serve. It also represents the differences found among EMS providers.

Brief Psychosocial History   A systematic gathering of an individual's current level of mental and social functioning.

Lethality Assessment   A systematic set of questions conducted in an effort to assess a person's determination to commit harm to themselves or harm to others.

Mental Status Exam   A full clinical work-up of a psychiatric patient including the assessment of overall psychiatric condition, diagnosis of existing disorders, prognosis, estimates of suitability for treatment of various kinds, formulation of overall personality, and compilation of historical and developmental data.

References

Davis, R. (2000). Cultural Health Care or Child Abuse? The Southeast Asian Practice of Cao Gio. *Journal American Academy of Nurse Practitioners.* 12(3), 89–95.

Hopper, J. (2007). *Child Abuse: Statistics, Research, and Resources.* Boston, MA: Harvard Medical School.

Thomas, J., & Woodall, S. J. (2006). *Responding to Psychological Emergencies: A Field Guide.* Clifton Park, NY: Thomson-Delmar Learning.

Fools Rush In

Psychosocial, Ethical, and Leadership Dimensions

- Safety
- Interagency Cooperation
- Team Dynamics
- Risk Management
- Internal and External Communication

Fools Rush In

The crew had been summoned to an emergency involving an injured person. Upon arrival, they found a large luxury home seemingly unoccupied. While walking up the long circle drive, they passed two men leaning on one of the high-dollar cars parked in the drive. While not leaving his position of repose, one of the men pointed to the front door and said, "In there." As is the custom, the crew quietly entered and called out "fire department!"

This veteran crew, composed of two firefighter/EMTs, an engineer/paramedic, and a captain/paramedic, were accustomed to making entry into unfamiliar places with uncertain circumstances. As they walked through the house with their EMS gear, it appeared as though every light in the house was on. They searched the first floor and continued to the stairs ascending to the second floor. They searched the upstairs bedrooms and also found nothing. The only room left was the plush master suite. Entering the room, they immediately realized that this was much more than an injured person.

On the white carpeted floor, next to the walk-in closet, lay a middle-aged woman in her nightgown. Her hands and legs were bound behind her back and her throat had been slashed from ear to ear. The blood loss was great and she was likely dead. Acting quickly, the paramedic and EMT placed the cardiac monitor on her and checked for other signs of life. The captain/paramedic immediately grabbed his portable radio and requested law enforcement.

Problem Solving

What Do You Know?

- Describe what you know about this incident.

What Do You Need to Know?

- What additional information is required before further decision making?

Resources

- What potential resources would be helpful at this stage?

Responsibilities

- What legal, ethical, organizational, or interpersonal responsibilities should you consider?

Action Plan

- Decide what you would do next if you were in this situation.

Justification of Your Action Plan

- Explain the rationale you used for your decision.

Follow-up

- Would your action plan require any follow-up? Why or why not?

The Rest of the Story

The victim was obviously dead. This was no longer an EMS scene; it was a crime scene. The crew, not knowing the dangerous nature of the call, had walked into a situation that could have proved fatal to any or all of them. The captain quickly notified dispatch to check on the ETA of the police department as the paramedic/engineer initiated a patch with the base hospital. After patching with the emergency department at the hospital and conferring with the physician, they removed the electrodes from the dead woman. They carefully exited the room taking special care not to disturb any potential evidence.

At this point, they still had not seen a police officer. When they reached the front door and started down the steps, it was evident why an officer had not made it up to the room. The two men they had passed on their way in were still leaning on the luxury car. However, now they were leaning, face down with their hands cuffed behind their backs.

Later in the evening, a police officer came to their station to get their statements and update them on the status of the murder. The two men were the family's chauffeur and mechanic. They were the prime suspects and were both in custody.

Discussion

- What role did complacency play in this scenario?
- What key safety standards were not followed?
- What is the lesson to be learned through this case study?
- In hindsight, how should this call been handled differently?

Skill Building

In the haste to respond and intervene, it is often easy to over-prioritize a sense of urgency. Time is our enemy, but by rushing in with little consideration regarding personal and scene safety, EMS responders run the risk of potential injury or death. This is often simplified as complacency, but it is quite possibly more than that. Occasionally, at the expense of safety, we focus only on the task at hand and skip some very important considerations. Those who are currently responders can probably relate to some, if not all, of the following risky behaviors:

- Entering an overturned vehicle before considering stabilizing the vehicle.
- Initiating patient care without donning the appropriate personal protective equipment (PPE).
- Not fastening seat belts.
- Not practicing strict lane accountability at intersections.
- Putting out a dumpster fire without a self-contained breathing apparatus (SCBA).
- The list goes on and on.

This crew had probably responded to many calls involving injured persons. Most of the time, these calls are routine and do not involve a murder. It is because of this that we can become complacent, letting our guard down. We expect each call to be as common and as routine as the last one. In this scenario, the captain failed to adequately assess scene safety. Don't fall victim to sacrificing safety in the name of urgency. Scene size-up is every crew member's job. Scene safety includes sizing up potential hazards, body substance isolation (BSI) precautions, using PPE, and removing patients from immediate danger (Thomas & Woodall, 2006). As you size up a scene, expect, and look for, the unexpected or the unusual.

In this case study, the captain could have done a better job assessing scene safety. He could have contacted the dispatch to see whether there was any further information. The two men in front of the house seemed rather calm. Typically, you would encounter an excited family member, neighbor, or friend. They also noticed that every light in the house was on. Should this have been interpreted to mean that something was wrong? Furthermore, the first floor was completely abandoned. Perhaps this is the point at which the captain should have checked for the ETA of the police department.

Scene safety requires the application of a specific assessment. Responders must constantly be aware of biohazards and take measures to assess and protect themselves through BSI precautions. Additionally, they must be fully aware of on-scene electrical hazards, traffic, structural instability, and a host of other dangerous challenges (Thomas & Woodall, 2006). Furthermore, scene safety is every team member's responsibility and all members should be looking for keys that indicate the possibility of the EMS or fire scene either being or becoming a crime scene. As is noted, scene safety is a dynamic and ongoing process and should be continuously evaluated and reevaluated. Our individual and team goal should be for every member on the team to return home safely after their shift. We are all responsible for the safety of those we work with. We are a team and the supervisor should always welcome another set of eyes and ears. When we let our guard down, we put ourselves and everyone whom we work with at risk.

Lessons Learned

What Do You Know?

A four-person Advanced Life Support (ALS) Engine Company was called to the scene of an "unknown medical-injured person." Upon arrival, they encountered two unknown individuals who directed them to the interior of the residence. The first floor of the residence was suspiciously vacant, and apparently every light in the house was on. As they searched the second floor, they found a middle-aged woman. She had been tied up and had lost a large volume of blood through a wound in her neck. She was deceased. The police department had not yet arrived on the scene.

What Do You Need to Know?

Critical information at this juncture would include finding out whether the police department had been dispatched and their ETA. It was no longer an EMS scene; it was now an active crime scene—active in that no law enforcement agency had interceded, the scene was not secured, and the identity and location of the perpetrator or perpetrators had not been established. In conjunction with ascertaining the status of the police department, the immediate safety concerns of the crew would need to be established.

Resources

After determining that the medical emergency scene was now the scene of an apparent murder, several potential resources become important. First, EMS protocol would require that every effort to save the woman's life should be initiated. If this was not possible and the patient was determined to be deceased, the crew's resource management strategy should adapt to the new situation. Had the patient been viable, further ALS assistance should be called and the dispatch of a medical helicopter should be considered. Second, in a situation of this magnitude, the captain/paramedic would want to call for the next level of supervision. The presence of a shift supervisor would provide an effective liaison to work with the police department on issues such as the crew's statement, evidence preservation, and chain-of-custody issues.

Responsibilities

The primary responsibility of a crew supervisor is the safety of the crew. The goal is often stated as "Everybody Goes Home." Crew safety is also an interpersonal and team responsibility. Each crew member should serve as the eyes and ears for every other member of the crew. This commitment to safety is manifested at many levels, from reminding each other to wear protective gloves when handling a patient to driving safety protocols, and in this case to recognizing that they have been called to the scene of a murder and their lives may be in danger.

Legally, the crew has a responsibility and role in the preservation of evidence. When working on the scene of a crime or potential crime, it is important that all crew members do their best to not disturb, move, or touch any potential evidence whenever possible. Attempting to practice sound evidence preservation will go a long way in building positive relationships with our law enforcement counterparts.

From the organizational perspective, adhering to standard operating procedures (SOPs) designed to enhance safety will assist in building and perpetuating a culture committed to individual and crew safety.

Action Plan

Action plans in dynamic situations such as this should be considered to be dynamic in nature. As the facts became known, the action plan would need to be quickly adapted. When it was determined that the patient was dead and had, likely, been murdered, crew safety would need to become the overriding concern. A rapid exit, keeping evidence preservation in mind, would become the top priority. Additionally, the urgent need of the police department should be conveyed via radio. Fortunately, the police department had arrived before the crew exited the residence. Had this not been the case, the crew should most definitely have not confronted, or questioned, anyone at the unsecured scene. Finally, the notification and request for the dispatch of the next level supervisor should be initiated.

Justification of Your Action Plan

Emergency medical providers are frequently called to scenes in which complete information is not available. In this scenario, it can be assumed that the murderers called 9-1-1 and stayed at the scene in hopes of diverting attention to themselves as suspects. This deception caused dispatch to provide inaccurate information to be passed on to the responding crew.

The on-scene EMS crew has the legal responsibility to preserve evidence; must follow EMS protocols and SOPs including running an EKG strip, patching with the base hospital, and contacting a supervisor; and should document what happened during this incident.

Follow-up

Follow-up in this case may involve a combined police/fire EMS critique. This critique could identify a need to enhance interagency cooperation directed at on-scene personnel safety, evidence preservation, and response sequence protocols in situations that may need to be secured before initiating rescue.

Summary

This case study graphically illustrates that the collective safety of all emergency responders calls for extensive interagency cooperation. The emergency response community cannot be safe and effective unless we know the needs, protocols, and mission of our fellow responders. This actual event illustrates just how fluid EMS scenes can be. Responders must take special care not to hyper-focus on their mission.

Team dynamics also comprise an important component of risk management. Risk management is not solely the responsibility of supervisors and managers. Each crew member has a responsibility to look out for potentially harmful actions or situations that might lead to the injury or death of their fellow crew members.

It all starts and ends with sound internal and external communication. On the internal level, this information exchange starts with the initial 9-1-1 call taker, to the dispatcher, to the supervisor, and then to the crew. It is during this process that all the pertinent questions need to be asked: Is the scene safe? Is the police department on scene? Are there any responsible parties on the scene that have been identified? On the external level, the EMS responder must be willing to, and effective at, communicating with other responding agencies. There is no such thing as a bad question as long as the question is conveyed in a constructive and professional manner.

Key Terms

BSI An acronym commonly used for body substance isolation that describes the actions taken by the EMS provider to ensure that those working with a patient are not unnecessarily exposed to the body substances emanating from a patient or patients.

Evidence Preservation A system of law enforcement protocols directed at preserving crime scene evidence when working at or on an active crime scene.

Personal Safety An individual's responsibility to practice procedurally driven safety precautions that are directed at enhancing the safety of each member.

PPE For EMS calls, this equipment is composed of latex gloves, eye protection, substance resistance pull-on sleeves, gowns, and filtering masks. In fire situations, PPE would consist of turnout gear, helmet, boots, and a SCBA.

Scene Safety   Procedures, protocols, and practices directed at determining whether, and ensuring that, a scene is safe for emergency response intervention. These considerations range from BSI to physical threats such as criminal activity in progress, to hazardous materials spills, to power lines down, and to any other circumstance that may prove harmful to emergency services personnel working at the scene (Thomas & Woodall, 2006).

References

Thomas, J., & Woodall, S. J. (2006). *Responding to Psychological Emergencies: A Field Guide.* Clifton Park, NY: Thomson-Delmar Learning.

Magnetic Personality

Psychosocial, Ethical, and Leadership Dimensions

- Customer Service
- Mental Illness

Magnetic Personality

Ambulance 49 was nearing the end of a busy shift. They had worked two codes, responded to a couple of motor vehicle accidents, and transported an intoxicated homeless woman to the emergency department for evaluation. While heading back to quarters to finish their paperwork, they were dispatched to a chest pain call. The information provided stated that the patient was a 33-year-old woman experiencing severe angina and shortness of breath. Turning on their lights and siren, they responded to an apartment building in an economically depressed neighborhood.

Upon arrival, they made their way up the elevator to a fourth-floor apartment. The door was ajar, so they went in announcing their presence with the loud call of "emergency medical services." The only person in the apartment was a woman who was on the couch watching television and smoking a cigarette. "Thank you for coming so fast," the woman said as she greeted the two paramedics.

"Someone here is experiencing chest pain?" one of the paramedics asked quizzically.

"Oh yes! I'm having problems with my heart," replied the woman in an anxious tone.

"How long have you been having this pain?" inquired the medic. At the same time, her partner was getting out the monitor and preparing the leads to take an EKG.

"Since this morning, after the visitors were here," came the reply.

"We're going to hook you up to this heart monitor and take a look," informed the second medic as he attached the leads. The monitor showed a normal sinus rhythm. The two medics proceeded to check her vital signs, which were also within the normal range.

"Your heart looks okay, can we check your lungs?" asked the first medic. After completing a thorough medical survey, the two medics were unable to find anything significant.

"Are you taking any medications?" queried the second medic.

"No," was the matter-of-fact reply.

"We can't seem to find anything wrong. Where does it hurt?"

"Right here," stated the woman as she put her hand over the center of her chest.

"Did something happen with your visitors this morning?" inquired the first medic.

"Yes, yes! They magnetized me and now my chest hurts!"

The two medics looked at each other with blank faces, neither one of them quite sure how to respond.

Problem Solving

What Do You Know?

- Describe what you know about this incident.

What Do You Need to Know?

- What additional information would be helpful before further decision making?

Resources

- What potential resources would be helpful at this stage?

Responsibilities

- What legal, ethical, organizational, or interpersonal responsibilities should you consider?

Action Plan

- Decide what you would do next if you were in this situation.

Justification of Your Action Plan

- Explain the rationale you used for your decision.

Follow-up

- Would your action plan require any follow-up? Why or why not?

▨▨▨▨▨ The Rest of the Story

After a lengthy pause, the second medic started nodding his head and said, "I understand. I know what to do." His partner just stood there uncertain about what was going to happen next. The medic put the pulse oximeter on his finger while explaining to the woman, "This machine measures a person's magnetic field. See my field is at 98 and that is normal." The woman nodded as he pulled out one of the defibrillator paddles. "I am going to wave this machine over your heart to demagnetize it." The woman nodded as he waived the paddles over her chest for several seconds. He then took the pulse oximeter off his finger and placed it on the woman's index finger. The display read 97.

"You're back to normal. That should take care of you for some time to come," informed the medic. His partner just smiled and nodded her head in agreement. "Do you think you need to go to the hospital?" asked the medic. "Oh no," responded the woman. "I feel just fine now."

"We just need you to sign this release form stating that you don't want to go to the hospital," stated the medic. The woman signed the form as the two paramedics gathered their gear. "Is there anything else we can do for you today?" asked the medic.

"No not today. Thank you both for your help," answered the woman.

The two paramedics picked up their gear and made their exit while wishing the woman a good evening.

Discussion

- Did this patient intervention violate any standard EMS protocols?
- Did the paramedics in this case do anything wrong?
- Should this patient have been transported for further evaluation?
- How would you document this call?
- Suggest some other strategies that these paramedics could have used with this patient.

Skill Building

Many times patients report symptoms that are not the result of physical problems. The patient in this case was suffering from the belief that she had been magnetized, and as a result, her heart had been affected. This is an example of delusional thinking. A delusion is a belief that is maintained even when there is a specific argument or data that would lead a reasonable person to abandon or reject the belief. Delusions are not always harmful; what may be a problem for some may be a source of comfort and deliverance for others. It is important to note that a belief that is commonly shared among a culture or a specific subculture cannot be considered a delusion. The manifestation of this woman's belief was chest pain, real or imagined.

If the woman was actually feeling chest pain, she may have been experiencing a hallucination. A hallucination is a perceptual experience with all the convincing properties of a real sensory experience. This perceptual experience exists even without the normal sensory stimulation required for that experience. In this case, the woman displayed no medical indicators that she should be experiencing chest pain, when in fact she really may have felt pain in her chest.

Delusions and hallucinations are seen as classic symptoms of a psychotic disorder. In this case, the two paramedics should have conducted a mental status exam. A mental status exam is an assessment of a patient's overall psychological condition. A good mental status exam includes an assessment of a person's physical appearance, speech, behavior, mood, and cognition or thought (Thomas & Woodall, 2006). A mental status exam is usually coupled with a lethality assessment to determine whether a patient is a danger to their self or to others.

The woman in this case appeared to be oriented. Her speech seemed to indicate that she was fully aware of what was happening to her. She was pleasant and cooperative. Even though she was delusional, she did not appear to be a danger to herself or to anyone else. A common mistake is to treat delusional thinking as a nonemergent problem.

The medics missed a critical factor by failing to ask the woman more questions about medications. The simple fact that she was taking, or had stopped taking, psychotropic medication could have indicated that the problem was more severe and that she needed to be evaluated by a mental health professional. It is also appropriate to inquire if a patient is seeing a psychologist or counselor. Had this been the case, the medics may have been able to call this provider and have them speak with the patient. This could help in getting a patient to agree to transport.

The medics in this case should be commended for their response to this woman's problems. The medic showed remarkable creativity and treated her with respect and dignity. Had the medics in this case argued with the woman about her delusional thinking and experience of chest pain, she might have become agitated and uncooperative. It is not the emergency medical service (EMS) provider's role to challenge or confront delusional thinking or hallucinations. This creative type of patient care is an example of good customer service. Had they transported her to "have her heart evaluated at the hospital," she likely would have received the mental health care she needs.

Lessons Learned

What Do You Know?

Ambulance 49 was dispatched on a call for a 33-year-old woman experiencing chest pain. Upon arrival, they discovered the woman to be fully alert and oriented, sitting on the couch watching television, and smoking a cigarette. After assessing the woman's vital signs and taking an electrocardiogram (EKG), the medics could not find any abnormal signs or symptoms. The woman denied taking any medications but did report that the problem began this morning after her visitors left. She further reported that the visitors had magnetized her, resulting in problems with her heart. One of the medics waived the defibrillator paddles over the woman to "demagnetize" her. He then used the pulse oximeter to show her that her "magnetic field" was back to normal.

What Do You Need to Know?

More information regarding the patient's psychosocial history would have been very helpful in this case. A psychosocial history would have revealed any history of mental illness, her emotional and behavioral history, her current level of mental and social functioning, as well as any family and social support systems she may have.

Resources

Information regarding this patient could have been gathered from a number of sources, including family, friends, neighbors, healthcare providers, and clergy. The sources of information could be identified by asking a question as simple as, "Is there anyone we can call to stay with you for an hour or so?" The medics could have also contacted their base hospital to see if she had ever been a patient there and if medical records were available. Some EMS systems are fortunate to have specialized responders who can work with mentally ill patients.

Responsibilities

Even in the absence of any physical symptoms, EMS responders are obligated to do a thorough medical exam. In the absence of medical signs or symptoms, it is wise to conduct a brief mental status exam accompanied by a brief psychosocial history and a lethality assessment. These assessments often reveal the presence of psychological symptoms that require treatment and/or intervention.

Action Plan

The medics in this case should have conducted a more comprehensive psychological exam and consulted with their base hospital.

Justification of Your Action Plan

Consulting with the base hospital would have covered the medics in the event that the woman called again later with the same complaint. Additionally, it is likely that the woman could ask another crew to "demagnetize" her in the future.

Follow-up

In this case, a referral to the community mental health agency or adult protective services might be advisable. The medics could have told her that they would have somebody stop by and check on her to see that she was doing okay. Given the fact that this patient was so cooperative and appreciative, she probably would have consented to this type of follow-up.

Summary

This case illustrates the fact that sometimes mental disorders are not viewed as being as serious or as emergent as medical problems. The danger with this type of thinking is that a serious problem can be missed or overlooked. Individuals with mental disorders often know when they are beginning to decompensate. Persons with mental illness are often lacking family and social support systems. If they are unsure about what to do or lack other resources, they may call 9-1-1 for assistance.

Many EMS providers receive a higher degree of training in the treatment of medical emergencies when compared with their training in the treatment of psychological emergencies. Because the EMS provider does not feel the same degree of proficiency in treating psychological emergencies, this can sometimes lead to a lower level of care. EMS providers should be aware that treating psychological emergencies is often more time consuming. It is the role of the EMS responder to ensure that these patients are connected with the components of the healthcare system that can give them the level of care that is required.

Key Terms

Decompensate   A term that describes the increasing severity of psychological symptoms accompanied by deterioration in mental and social functioning.

Delusion   A belief that is maintained in spite of argument, data, and refutation that should (reasonably) be sufficient to destroy it.

Hallucination   A perceptual experience with all the compelling subjective properties of a real sensory impression but without the normal physical stimulus for that sensory modality.

Lethality Assessment   A systematic set of questions conducted in an effort to assess a person's determination to commit harm to themselves or harm to others.

Mental Status Exam   A full clinical work-up of a psychiatric patient including the assessment of overall psychiatric condition, diagnosis of existing disorders, prognosis, estimates of suitability for treatment of various kinds, formulation of overall personality, and compilation of historical and developmental data.

Psychosocial History   A systematic gathering of an individual's psychological history, emotional and behavioral history, family and social supports, and current level of mental and social functioning.

Psychotic Disorder   Often used to describe a set of symptoms characterized by delusional thinking and/or hallucinations.

References

Thomas, J., & Woodall, S. J. (2006). *Responding to Psychological Emergencies: A Field Guide*. Clifton Park, NY: Thomson-Delmar Learning.

You Did What?

Psychosocial, Ethical, and Leadership Dimensions

- Interpersonal Skills
- Interagency Cooperation
- Incident Command

You Did What?

"Ambulance 244 respond to a motor vehicle accident," blared the rig radio. The two-person ALS ambulance crew quickly rinsed the remaining soap from the sides of the rig, acknowledged their response, and hit the street heading for 4400 Oak Street. As the first responders on the scene, the senior paramedic sized up the situation. The wreck was serious with several victims in and out of the two vehicles involved. The senior paramedic grabbed the radio and gave an on-scene report, requesting additional resources, including another ALS ambulance and the fire department.

After relaying the benchmark information to dispatch, the senior paramedic provided her action report. "Ambulance 244 will assume Oak Street command, initiating triage and treatment." Their hands were full with one immediate patient, two delayed patients, and several minor patients who would be assessed and treated as time allowed. The senior paramedic initiated treatment on the immediate patient, enlisting the assistance of a police officer and a self-described EMT bystander. The second paramedic started the assessment on one of the delayed patients.

For what seemed an eternity, the two paramedics worked as fast and proficiently as they could. Some 10 minutes into the call, no additional resources had arrived. Within hearing distance of a police officer holding an IV (intravenous) bag, the senior paramedic sighed, "Man, where are those guys? I need some help and I need it now."

"Oh, I heard your report but saw everyone walking around and thought it wasn't too serious," the police officer stated. "So I canceled everyone else. Sorry."

Problem Solving

What Do You Know?

- Describe what you know about this incident.

What Do You Need to Know?

- What additional information is required before further decision making?

Resources

- What potential resources would be helpful at this stage?

Responsibilities

- What legal, ethical, organizational, or interpersonal responsibilities should you consider?

Action Plan

- Decide what you would do next if you were in this situation.

Justification of Your Action Plan

- Explain the rationale you used for your decision.

Follow-up

- Would your action plan require any follow-up? Why or why not?

The Rest of the Story

Probably due to the stress of the moment and having had a history of poor working relations with this jurisdiction's police department, the senior paramedic went ballistic. She shouted, "You did what!! I am the medical control on this scene! Never ever consider messing with my resources unless you confer with me first! Your actions may cost at least one of these patients their life! It's a good thing that you at least can serve as an IV pole or I'd run you off my scene." This led the police officer to get his sergeant, the sergeant to get the lieutenant, and the lieutenant to file a complaint with the emergency medical service agency. The complaint came to the director of operations who notified the senior paramedic's supervisor. The senior paramedic acknowledged her actions and was eventually reprimanded for her inappropriate outburst.

Discussion

- What were the incident command responsibilities of the senior paramedic and the police officer on this scene?
- Did the senior paramedic do anything wrong?
- Did the officer on the scene do anything wrong?
- What may have led to this tactical and communication breakdown?
- What measures could be taken to ensure that this would not happen again?
- Did the senior paramedic's actions solve the immediate problem?
- How could this have been handled better?

Skill Building

In the field setting, it is necessary for EMS, fire, and law enforcement to work together. In most cases, this is accomplished by compartmentalizing an incident according to the functions and duties of each responding agency. It is important for each emergency responding agency to understand each agency's mission. This can be accomplished only through pre-incident training focused on interagency mission clarification and cooperation. Scenes often provide multiple challenges. Calls involving driving under the influence (DUI) of drugs or alcohol, with injuries, gunshot wounds, stabbings, and crimes involving domestic violence represent just a few instances in which the law enforcement mission and the emergency medical mission intersect. By interfacing with those agencies you respond with, you will learn their mission, roles, and responsibilities.

The senior paramedic in this scenario technically did not do anything wrong. The seriousness of the call created urgency in her mind and she lost her temper. The police officer who canceled her resources was clearly wrong, but he should have been treated in a respectful and professional manner. This call definitely deserves a multiagency critique and represents a great opportunity to learn the roles, responsibilities, and mission of each agency involved.

Law enforcement officers are often thrust into support roles in emergency medical scenes. They can be, and most often are, handy and helpful, but they have responsibilities to fulfill as well. This situation could have most easily been avoided through clear understanding of the incident command system (ICS) and the roles and responsibilities of all agencies involved.

The senior paramedic was unprofessional in publicly dressing-down the police officer. She more than likely made a difficult working relationship even worse. Her angry reaction to the canceling of the resources she was expecting did not, in any way, alleviate the situation. The patients would have been better served if she had simply got on the radio and requested the necessary resources again. After the patients had been transported, she most definitely should pull the officer aside and professionally discuss the importance of understanding each agency's role. This would strengthen her relationship with the officer and his agency and serve to prohibit this type of action from recurring.

Lessons Learned

What Do You Know?

An ALS ambulance crew arrived on the scene of a serious motor vehicle accident (MVA), initiated triage and treatment, and called for additional emergency medical assistance, including the fire department. After waiting for a considerable amount of time, the senior paramedic wondered out loud about why the additional resources she requested had not yet arrived on the scene. When a police officer informed her that he had canceled those resources, she became irate, creating a considerable scene.

What Do You Need to Know?

It would be helpful to know whether it is a common practice in this jurisdiction for law enforcement to contact fire/EMS dispatch and cancel or reconfigure EMS resources already dispatched to an emergency scene. If this was a common practice, this occurrence could be viewed as a systemic versus individual problem. All EMS responders must know, understand, and be able to utilize the incident command system.

Resources

Additional resources would need to be re-dispatched to the scene. In the interim, the on-scene crew would need to continue triage and serve those most seriously injured first. It would also be wise to place a medical helicopter on standby or to have them immediately dispatched if they would arrive before the additional land-based resources.

Responsibilities

From an interpersonal perspective, the senior paramedic had a professional responsibility to interact with the police officer in a professional manner while on scene and in the public's eye.

Chewing someone out in public, even when that person is obviously in the wrong, does not serve the best interest of the patients, her professional interest, her agency's interest, and/or the interests of the police officer and the agency he represents.

Action Plan

In this case, the damage has already been done. First and foremost, the resources were canceled and must be re-dispatched. It would be prudent to include a command presence on this scene. Through the early implementation of the incident command system, the paramedic involved in directly rendering treatment would have been able to focus on her patient. An incident commander would be monitoring the response of additional assistance and may have been able to intercept the order to cancel other responding resources. This could be accomplished even while the incident commander was in route to the scene. Treatment of the injured must continue to the best extent possible considering the current on-scene resources. Finally, the verbal altercation of the police officer should stop immediately. The paramedic had vented and a return to professional interactions would best serve the injured. After the scene has been terminated and all the victims have been treated and transported, the two agencies should get together for a brief and professional discussion of what went wrong on this scene and how it can be avoided in the future. It would be a good idea for each agency to request a higher level of supervision if supervisors were already on the scene. These higher-level supervisors could mediate the post-emergency critique, act as a calming influence, and suggest higher-order solutions in an effort to avoid this type of situation in the future.

Justification of Your Action Plan

The action plan in this scenario is pretty straightforward. The resources that were requested and canceled should be re-dispatched. Rapidly establishing an incident command cannot be overemphasized. It is difficult to be involved in patient treatment and also meet the requirements of a sound incident command. The treatment of the injured must be continued with the available resources until additional assistance arrives. The negative interpersonal exchange must be placed on the back burner until the situation is successfully mitigated. The importance of professional interactions and adherence to each agency's protocols should be addressed while both agencies involved remain on the scene. In instances in which interagency conflict arise, it is always a good idea to seek the assistance of higher levels of supervision.

Follow-up

In a case such as this where patient care is compromised, it is always advisable to file a written report. Although it would be unfortunate, it is entirely possible that the actions of the police officer could have attributed to a less than desirable patient outcome. If this was, in fact, the case, considerable liability could be at issue. Hopefully, this would not be the case and patient outcomes would not have been affected. However, written documentation of this incident could also lead to actions directed at ensuring that this would not happen again.

Summary

The need to successfully interact with other emergency response agencies is a reality. Understanding the roles, responsibilities, and mission of other emergency response services will better enable all parties involved to work together effectively, increasing interagency cooperation, in the interest of those we serve. In the urgency frequently found on an emergency scene adherence to agency protocols can sometimes be overlooked. An effective and strong incident command system can assist all involved in making sure that an incident runs smoothly and important benchmarks are not overlooked.

We should all seek to improve our interpersonal communication skills. The need for professionalism on the emergency scene is a requirement that those working on the emergency scene should constantly be cognizant of. Tone, place, and professionalism are all important considerations when interacting with fellow emergency responders.

Key Terms

DUI   driving under the influence of drugs or alcohol. The legal blood alcohol limits are defined individually by each state.

Incident Command System   A structured incident management system that is commonly employed at incidents in which span-of-control is an issue. The presence of an incident commander allows those treating the patients to focus on the task level, whereas the incident commander directs attention to strategy, safety, and resource management issues such as hospital and patient transportation availability.

Triage   The medical protocol–driven process in which multiple patients are assessed as to the seriousness and level of treatment required. Those with life-threatening injuries are the first to be treated and transported. Those with serious injuries that are not life threatening are the second to be treated and transported and those with minor injuries are the last to be treated and transported.

7

It'll Only Take a Minute

Psychosocial, Ethical, and Leadership Dimensions

- Ethics
- Standard Operating Procedures
- Team Dynamics

▨▨▨ It'll Only Take a Minute

"Hey, I was out late last night and didn't have a chance to feed the horses. Could we drive out to my place so they won't go hungry? I think they need some water too."

Greg had heard this many times before from Joe, his senior paramedic partner, and was really getting fed up. "Here we go again!" he thought to himself. He really didn't like being placed in these types of situations but was finding little trips and stops like this to be more the norm than the exception. He was still the new guy expecting to complete his probationary year in a few months and didn't want to make trouble. By the same token, he didn't want to get in trouble either.

Greg really respected Joe, and since they had been working together, Greg had learned a great deal. Both of them live in the same small town and Joe had an outstanding reputation as a "heads-up" paramedic. Joe's ranch was in their response area, but it was at the far end of it and made for a very poor response time to the other side of the district. He knew it was time to say something and decided to give it a try. "You know Joe, I'm not really comfortable going out to the ranch all the time while we're on duty. We leave the west end of our district without coverage and I just think we should stay more central," Greg pleaded.

"Come on Greg," Joe replied, shaking his head. "This will only take a minute and besides it doesn't happen all the time. If the company paid me what I'm worth I could hire some help for the days I'm on, but you and I both know that's not going to happen. Sit tight I can make up the response time with my great driving ability."

"Well, you're the boss," was all Greg had to say.

Problem Solving

What Do You Know?

- Describe what you know about this incident.

What Do You Need to Know?

- What additional information would be helpful before further decision making?

Resources

- What potential resources would be helpful at this stage?

Responsibilities

- What legal, ethical, organizational, or interpersonal responsibilities should you consider?

Action Plan

- Decide what you would do next if you were in this situation.

Justification of Your Action Plan

- Explain the rationale you used for your decision.

Follow-up

- Would your action plan require any follow-up? Why or why not?

The Rest of the Story

After the 10-minute drive to the ranch, Joe jumped out and headed for the barn. Sitting in the rig and monitoring the radio, Greg could see Joe through the loft door chucking hay down to his two horses. He had just glanced away when he heard a loud yell.

"My leg! My leg! I think I've broke my ankle! Greg hurry! Come, help! Quick!"

Greg jumped from the rig and ran to the barn finding Joe flat on his back at the foot of the loft ladder. "Darn Greg! I slipped off the ladder and I think I may have broken my ankle. It may just be a bad sprain but it's already swelling. Go get me some tape and a cold pack."

Greg obediently went into action, returning to the rig to retrieve the items Joe requested. "Thanks Greg," Joe replied as Greg handed him the tape and bent down to help.

"Yeah, I'm going to tape this baby up to restrict the swelling and get the cold pack on it."

As he observed the ankle with the boot off, Greg saw just how serious the injury was. "Man Joe, this is going to require an X-ray."

"No way," Joe abruptly stated. "I'm going to be just fine. As a matter of fact, after I get this fixed up we're heading back to quarters to wash the rig. I feel a big slip and fall on the wet driveway coming on."

"What do you mean," Joe stated sensing a serious problem.

"Greg, I don't have any sick leave left and I can't afford to be off without pay. You've got to understand and work with me on this. I've been around a lot longer than you and I know this will work without a hitch."

Discussion

- Is it OK to take care of personal business at your home or locations other than the station or quarters while on duty?
- What will Joe's plan to fake an injury constitute?
- Is this a legal issue or an ethical issue?
- If they follow through with Joe's plan, is Greg guilty of anything?
- Could Greg have done anything earlier in his working relationship with Joe that might have possibly kept things from getting to the point reached in this scenario?

Skill Building

Many EMS and fire responders work a version of a 12 or 24-hour shift. This schedule makes it very difficult to run errands such as going to the bank, picking up dry cleaning, and returning library books. It is not unusual for fire and emergency medical service (EMS) responders to attempt to complete a few personal tasks, providing that their needs don't interfere with response times and readiness to respond. Crews wishing to run errands while on duty must take several things into consideration before they embark on such excursions:

- What is my agency's policy regarding such activities?
- How do my immediate supervisors feel about these activities?
- How will running errands on duty and in service be perceived by the general public?
- Should my partner or my crew have a discussion of what is and what is not acceptable? How could such a discussion help in the overall morale of a crew or partnership?

Joe is contemplating workers compensation fraud. The workers compensation insurance fund is monies set aside for employees injured at work. It was felt that if a worker was injured while working for someone else, the injured party is not required to use his or her personally accrued sick leave. Fraudulently filing a workers compensation claim is a serious crime and is committed in the workplace so frequently that investigating it requires a tremendous amount of costly resources. Because Joe stated that he didn't have any paid sick leave on the books, he was basically telling Greg that he was going to seek workers compensation. Had Greg gone along with Joe's plan, he would also be culpable. Greg is also on probation and would more than likely lose his job should an investigation result.

The general population knows that EMS and fire services are available 365 days a year and 24 hours a day, but more than likely they don't know how these services are staffed. When they see uniformed personnel running personal errands while on duty, they may not be able to empathize with our actions. They know that they are not allowed to run personal errands while they are at work, and if they are aware of the shift schedules of fire and EMS, they still may very well feel compelled to report their observations to an agency head or local politician.

When groups of people are required to work together, it is always a good idea to have a discussion that sets the boundaries of acceptable actions and behaviors for the group. The best place to start is with the agency's policies and procedures. If you work under a governing body, you would also want to consult the administrative regulations laid down by that group. Policies, procedures, and administrative regulations will normally not cover every detail. Therefore, it will be up to the EMS crew's designated supervisor or the company officer on the fire/EMS truck to set the tone and explain his or her expectations of the crew. Crew members should have a say and this is a good time to clarify any questions or concerns. Many issues that arise are not necessarily prohibited by formal written policies, procedures, or administrative regulations. These issues fall into a category referred to as ethics.

Ethics can be defined as the study and evaluation of human conduct in light of moral principles. Moral principles may be viewed either as the standard of conduct that individuals have constructed for themselves or as the body of obligations and duties that a particular society requires of its members.

Lessons Learned

What Do You Know?

Greg and Joe have been working together on the ambulance for some time. Greg is a new paramedic and has really benefited from Joe's tutelage. While on duty, Joe frequently drives the ambulance out to his ranch to care for his horses. Although his ranch lies within their response area, it is at the far east end. Greg has become increasingly uncomfortable with this and let it be known to Joe. Despite Greg's objections, Joe convinces him to go to the ranch.

After feeding his horses, Joe fell from the loft ladder severely injuring his ankle. Greg assists him and recommends he seek medical treatment. Joe explains that he is out of sick leave and suggests a plan to make it look like he fell while they were washing the ambulance.

What Do You Need to Know?

Greg should be aware of his company's policies regarding running personal errands while on duty. There are also likely to be policies about first due response areas and where emergency response vehicles are allowed to be in that area. Additionally, every employee should know the procedures for reporting on-the-job injuries.

In this particular case, Greg should consider the fact that it is illegal to falsely claim workers compensation benefits. Many employers hire private investigators to look into the veracity of a claim if they suspect fraud. Workers compensation fraud is a felony. Conviction can result in prison sentences and large fines.

Resources

Greg should consult the policy manual regarding the proper action to take.

Responsibilities

Every EMS professional has the responsibility to follow their agency's policies and procedures. Failure to do so frequently results in disciplinary action. They also have the responsibility to follow the law. EMS professionals are held to a higher standard and are expected to be model citizens when it comes to following the law.

Ethically, Greg and Joe have to ask themselves what is the right thing to do. Joe must consider how his actions will impact Greg. Greg is a probationary employee and Joe is asking him to commit a felony. Greg must consider how his actions will impact his career and his family.

Lastly, both of them have the responsibility to maintain the public's trust of the EMS profession. Although the public may be a little more forgiving of an EMS professional taking care of his horses, a jury is less likely to be forgiving in the case of workers compensation fraud. By committing the crime of fraud, Joe and Greg do damage to the reputation of EMS providers everywhere.

Action Plan

Greg should insist that Joe report the incident truthfully. If Joe refuses to do this, Greg should request to speak with his supervisor and should immediately document what took place.

Justification of Your Action Plan

Greg is a probationary employee; as such he can be dismissed from his position for any reason. The risk to his future in EMS and to his family is too great to participate in the commission of a crime. Joe may be out of sick leave and may face the possibility of time of without pay, but he will still have a job to come back to. Many agencies are able to find light-duty assignments for employees who are injured both on and off the job. Joe and Greg may face disciplinary action for taking care of personal business while on duty; however, the penalties for this will be far less severe than any possible sentence from a felony conviction.

Follow-up

The company's management is likely to follow up this incident by conducting an investigation. Joe and Greg need to be honest and cooperate with the investigation. There is a possibility that Joe may have some hard feelings as a result of Greg's insistence on following procedures. Even though Greg did the right thing, both of them should discuss this with each other after the investigation is complete and make every effort to resolve any hard feelings. Conflict between team members can sometimes lead to decreased levels of performance that in turn have the potential to impact patient care and safety.

Summary

Almost every individual makes mistakes in their life, and almost every employee makes mistakes at work. When this happens, the wise thing to do is to take responsibility for your actions and learn from the mistake. Sometimes people look for a way to cover-up their mistakes. Although this may seem like a way to prevent detection, history is full of examples of individuals who made their situations far worse by trying to cover-up their initial mistakes. In the end, we are far more likely to come out ahead if we own up to our mistakes and accept whatever the consequence may be.

This case is a good example of how one team member's actions can place every other team member at risk. Joe should have given more thought to how his trips to the ranch could impact Greg, particularly because Greg is still in his probationary period. Every team member needs to be aware that they have the responsibility to take care of their team members. Too often this view is limited to issues such as patient care and safety. In many ways, individual success is related to team success. Each team member has the responsibility to see that the other team members are following policies and procedures, following the law, and maintaining a high standard of professional ethics.

Key Terms

Workers Compensation   Insurance to cover medical care and compensation for employees who are injured in the course of performing their job.

Ethics   The ability to make sound decisions based on what is considered right and wrong, what is morale, and what is legal.

Light Duty   Reassignment of an employee to another position, compatible with medically imposed restrictions and/or limitations.

8

Why at 3 am?

Psychosocial, Ethical, and Leadership Dimensions

- Customer Service
- Patient Advocacy
- Interpersonal Skills

Why at 3 am?

The ladder crew at a suburban fire station was feeling tired from a busy day of running calls. They had been on a number of EMS calls and one dumpster fire. There had been no time to shop, so dinner became another one of those fast-food experiences. They were hoping for a quiet night. Unfortunately, this was not to be the case.

At 11 pm, they were dispatched to a motor vehicle accident requiring extrication. The call took just under an hour. They had to extricate the patient and provide treatment for deep lacerations to both knees. The patient was stable and was transferred to the ambulance for transport. Feeling good about the successful rescue, the crew headed back to the station looking forward to getting some sleep.

At 3:14 am, the tones went off dispatching them to another call: "Ill person, Rock River subdivision." Rock River is an active adult community that they had been to three times earlier in the shift. They responded with lights and siren to a private residence in that community. The mobile computer terminal advised that the patient was a 58-year-old male complaining of a headache. One crew member made the comment that he was the one with a headache due to lack of sleep. This bit of humor broke the tension and lightened the crew's mood as they responded to the call.

They arrived at the residence and were escorted to the master bedroom by the patient's wife. The two EMTs began assessing the patient. The paramedic captain started interviewing the patient and getting a history. The patient complained that he had been experiencing "a really bad headache for the past three days." When the captain asked him why he called the fire department, he replied "I just can't stand it anymore." The patient further stated, "I thought about calling you this afternoon, but I didn't want to bother you guys."

The EMTs found that his vital signs were normal and that there were no visible signs of head trauma. Both pupils were normal and reactive. The patient denied any type of blunt impact to the head or the use of any substances. The patient indicated that he had been treating himself with Tylenol but that it had "stopped working." The patient's wife confirmed his story. After hearing this story, one member of the crew started shaking his head from left to right and walked out of the room.

The captain politely told the patient that they could find nothing wrong with him other than his headache. He asked the patient what he would like them to do for him. The patient then stated, "I know that you have drugs with you. Can't you just give me something stronger so I can just get some sleep?" At this time, the ambulance crew arrived.

Problem Solving

What Do You Know?

- Describe what you know about this incident.

What Do You Need to Know?

- What additional information is required before further decision making?

Resources

- What potential resources would be helpful at this stage?

Responsibilities

- What legal, ethical, organizational, or interpersonal responsibilities should you consider?

Action Plan

- Decide what you would do next if you were in this situation.

Justification of Your Action Plan

- Explain the rationale you used for your decision.

Follow-up

- Would your action plan require any follow-up? Why or why not?

The Rest of the Story

The captain made contact with the base hospital and consulted with the physician on duty. The physician recommended that the patient be transported to the emergency department. The captain relayed the physician's recommendation and the patient became noticeably agitated. He stated, "All the doctor and the hospital want is my money. Are you sure you just can't give me something for this darn headache?" The captain gently informed the man that he could not do that without a doctor's order and that he would need to be examined in the emergency department. Because money seemed to be an issue, the captain also informed the patient that his wife could drive him to the hospital emergency department, avoiding the ambulance charge, so that he could be checked out.

The patient's wife agreed and encouraged him to "go get checked." After discussing this for 5 minutes, the man finally consented to transport by ambulance. However, he insisted on getting dressed, using the rest room, and getting a drink of water before he left. The engine company and the ambulance crew waited for 15 minutes while he got ready.

Discussion

- Why do you think he waited until 3 am to call 9-1-1?
- Did this crew provide the best possible service?
- Did the crew member who walked out of the room shaking his or her head do anything wrong?
- What will you do differently when you are the one becoming frustrated?
- What steps could your agency initiate to help emergency responders prevent and manage this type of frustration?

Skill Building

Calls like this often happen in the middle of the night because that is when people feel most alone and vulnerable. The man in this case may have been unable to sleep for several nights and his inability to sleep this night may have been what pushed him over the edge. People have fewer resources when they are experiencing a crisis in the middle of the night. They are reluctant to wake up family, friends, or neighbors. Older adults oftentimes have difficulty driving at night. So what do they do? They call 9-1-1. They believe, and rightly so, that it is our job to respond when they are having an emergency.

Many times emergency service personnel become frustrated when they do not perceive the call to be a true emergency. This is especially true when these calls come at mealtime or in the middle of the night. The crew in this case had been running all day. They may have just gotten to sleep after the car wreck when this call was dispatched. Clearly, they were tired. In the back of their minds, they were all probably debating with themselves on whether it would be worth it to go back to bed when they got back to the station. Undoubtedly, their patience was wearing thin and they were becoming frustrated. Although they may have felt frustrated, emergency responders are not allowed to let those feelings manifest themselves during patient interactions. It is important to remember that every person deserves the same degree of customer service regardless of the time of day (Brunacini, 1996). To the credit of this crew, they handled the situation very well. The crew member who went outside may have done the right thing, providing that the remaining crew did not need his assistance. Had he remained, he may have verbally or physically demonstrated his frustration. When appropriate, he would probably be wise to discuss his actions with his captain.

The problem of sleep deprivation is a serious concern among emergency responders. Sleep deprivation can lead to critical errors in driving, safety, and patient care. Chronic sleep deprivation can lead to long-term health problems (Pellin, 2003), increased use of sick leave, and more on-the-job injuries (Dement, 2002). Emergency medical services (EMS) agencies can increase the health and wellness of their employees by being aware of sleep needs versus the amount of sleep their people are getting. Many agencies allow their employees to nap in the middle of the day. This allows them to recuperate and revitalize, so that they remain sharp throughout the rest of the shift.

Lessons Learned

What Do You Know?

A tired crew has been dispatched to an ill person call at 3:14 am. Upon arrival, they encountered an older gentleman complaining of a severe headache that had lasted over the last three days. The patient assessment indicated no other significant findings. After the assessment, the crew and the hospital physician recommended that he should go to the emergency department for further assessment and treatment. The patient initially balked at going to the emergency department, but after some convincing by the crew and his wife, he relinquished.

What Do You Need to Know?

Additional information about the patient's health history would be helpful. Had he previously been treated for migraines or severe headaches? Had he ever had a traumatic brain injury? Had he recently changed his caffeine intake? Does he have any family history of cancer? Questions along these lines would prove beneficial in getting to a more definitive identification of the potential causes of his headaches.

Resources

The patient's wife proved to be a valuable resource as she convinced him to go to the emergency department for further evaluation and treatment. Family members represent a key component of most individuals' support system. Patients will frequently comply with the advice provided by a family member. An additional resource can often be a fellow crew member. A good team leader knows the strengths and weaknesses of each team member and calls on them for special assistance when their particular skill set meets the requirements of a given situation.

Responsibilities

When examining what could have potentially gone wrong on this call, it is necessary to emphasize that leaving this patient with what he described as a severe headache could, and probably would, constitute patient abandonment. As certified EMS personnel, we have an ethical obligation to serve as patient advocates until such time that the emergency is addressed, the patient is satisfied, and the patient either signs a medical release or is transported to a higher level of care.

Organizationally and interpersonally, we have the responsibility to facilitate positive patient encounters, delivering expeditious, competent, and professional care. We do this in the interest of those we serve, our agency, and our personal satisfaction for a job well done.

Action Plan

This incident, although requiring some special attention and extra patience, reached a successful outcome. The chief complaint was assessed and the patient was transported for further evaluation and treatment. Utilizing the approach that this crew did would prove to be a sound course of action.

Justification of Your Action Plan

If an action plan similar to the actions taken by this ladder crew was implemented, it would be fully justified. The outcome was successful and positive and everyone parted company on a satisfied basis. Additionally, all medical protocols were met, and a sound and thorough assessment was performed. This was a close call and could have easily degraded into a bad experience for all involved. Fortunately, it did not. By spending the extra time and being attentive to the patient's needs, they were able to convince the patient to be transported. EMS field responders do not have the skill and all the necessary diagnostic tools required to make definitive field diagnosis. This patient may have had a brain bleed or other serious medical problem that could only be assessed, diagnosed, and treated in the hospital setting.

Follow-up

The supervisor of this crew would most certainly want to follow-up with the crew member who went to the truck rather than participating in a frustrating call. It is more than likely that the crew member would not have left his crew understaffed had this been a call of a more serious nature. However, the importance of total team continuity and teamwork would need to be reinforced by the supervisor.

Summary

There are times when we all become frustrated. The mark of a professional is how these frustrations are handled. When you encounter patients and situations that test your patience be prepared and mask these emotions while attending the patient. Your attitude and professionalism not only reflect your personal professionalism but also reflect on your crew and your agency. We must also be constantly aware that we serve as patient advocates. An advocate serves in a person's best interest in situations in which that person lacks the knowledge or does not have the physical ability to serve as their own advocate. This is what we do, whether 3 am or 3 pm, whether the patient is conscious or unconscious, even when we are tired.

Our interpersonal skills and our ability to utilize those skills in situations of great urgency and in situations that simply test our patience determine whether a patient/customer encounter will be a positive or negative one. Maintaining our role as the patient advocate will most always lead to excellent customer service.

Key Terms

Sleep Deprivation   Being deprived of adequate quality sleep or an extended period. The negative impacts of sleep deprivation are cumulative in nature and can lead to long-term health problems as well as increasing the probability of accidents and injuries (Dement, 1991).

Customer Service   The process and practice of delivering services. From the fire/EMS and EMS perspective, this is usually defined as the manner in which services are delivered that produces a positive outcome.

Patient Advocacy   The act of assuming the role of a patient representative in circumstances in which the patient is unwilling or unable to serve in his or her best interest regarding treatment, transportation, and medical care.

Interpersonal Skills   Those skills and abilities that allow a person to successfully interact with others.

References

Brunacini, A. (1996). *Essentials of Fire Department Customer Service*. Stillwater, OK: Fire Protection Publications Oklahoma State University.

Dement, W. (1991). *What All Undergraduates Should Know About How Their Sleeping Lives Affect Their Working Lives*. Palo Alto, CA: Stanford University Press.

Dement, W. (2002). And So to Bed. *Economist* 365(8304).

Pellin, Z. (2003). Sleep Deprivation Affects Immune Cells. *Sleep Medicine* 4(5).

Where Do We Go from Here?

Psychosocial, Ethical, and Leadership Dimensions

- Customer Service
- EMS Protocols
- Standard Operating Procedures
- Supervision
- Teamwork

Where Do We Go from Here?

The one-year-old baby was not doing well. The young mother was trying to get the feverish, coughing, croupy infant home after a long day of work. The baby was fighting the car seat and literally screaming in discomfort and frustration. "I can't handle this," she said out loud. Since she had no cell phone, she started looking for a pay phone.

She ended up at a convenience market and asked the clerk to call 9-1-1.

It was just about 10 pm; lights-out time and the paramedic engine company was preparing for what they hoped would be a full night of uninterrupted sleep.

"Channel 2 EMS assignment—ill infant. Engine 11; Ambulance 14. At the Quicky Mart; 14th street and Highway 9."

"Here we go again! Man, I was just about in the rack," complained the captain/ EMT.

In a few short minutes, they rolled into the market and grabbed the EMS gear. They checked inside and the clerk pointed to an old beat-up foreign model car in the parking lot.

The woman had stepped out of the car and the firefighter/paramedic met her beside the car. "You called about an ill baby," he inquired.

"Yes, I was trying to get her home but I just got too worried. I think she needs to go to the hospital."

"Let us take a look," the firefighter/paramedic said in a soothing voice. "Wow mom, she is hot to the touch and sounds pretty croupy. We better take her to the hospital. Where do you want her to go?"

"Well I live up by West Regional Hospital. It would be great if I could get her close to home. My car is not running great so I hate to go too far," she replied.

"Ma'am, I think she should go to Central Children's Hospital. They are well equipped to handle little ones," the firefighter/paramedic replied. About that time, the ambulance arrived and the crew persuaded the mother to get on the gurney and hold the baby while the assessment continued. Once the mother and child were secured in the back of the ambulance, the firefighter/paramedic pulled the captain aside and said, "Skip, I wouldn't take my dog to West Regional. I know it is closer but I just hate that hospital and Central is a children's hospital."

Problem Solving

What Do You Know?

- Describe what you know about this incident.

What Do You Need to Know?

- What additional information is required before further decision making?

Resources

- What potential resources would be helpful at this stage?

Responsibilities

- What legal, ethical, organizational, or interpersonal responsibilities should you consider?

Action Plan

- Decide what you would do next if you were in this situation.

Justification of Your Action Plan

- Explain the rationale you used for your decision.

Follow-up

- Would your action plan require any follow-up? Why or why not?

The Rest of the Story

The baby was eventually transported to Central Children's Hospital, even though the captain/EMT expressed her disagreement with the decision. She made a mental note to discuss her feelings with the fire-fighter/paramedic when the time was appropriate.

Upon arriving in quarters and while restocking the truck, she de-cided to let her thoughts be known. "Sam, I know you're a paramedic and I'm just an EMT. I respect your certification, your judgment, and your skills in almost every call that we've been on together, but in my opinion that baby was not stable enough to make the long trip to Cen-tral Children's. By taking her there we basically forced her to take a much longer ride than to West Regional."

"But Skip, you know as well as I do that West Regional is a dump. You're a mom. Would you want your child taken there?" he replied.

"Probably not; but you chose to ignore our EMS protocols, which require us to take an unstable patient to the closest appropriate hos-pital. We prolonged the time it would take to have her evaluated by a higher medical authority—a physician."

Discussion

- Were any EMS protocols violated in this scenario?
- What role does our personal preference play in making field-based decisions?
- Did it matter that the mother wanted to have her child taken to West Regional?
- Had the outcome been negative, what personal and organiza-tional liability did the firefighter/paramedic expose himself and the organization to?
- What kinds of problems can arise when an EMT supervises a paramedic?

Skill Building

Failure to transport an unstable patient to the closest appropriate hospital may be a serious breach of protocol. Establishing patient stability or in-stability represents a variable within the equation that is often difficult to determine. That's why we have the ability to contact the base emergency department and seek the advice of a physician. The decisions of the base hospital physician are predicated on the picture that is painted by the paramedic or emergency medical technician (EMT) giving the report.

Problems arise when we allow our personal opinions and/or biases to cloud our judgment. At times, it is necessary to trust the system and place our personal feelings aside. This is an effective way in which to manage our personal liability and that of the agency. We are members of the greater emergency medical service (EMS) system and should be committed to play by the rules. In this case, the mother wanted to transport her child to a facility closer to her home. Given her explanation about her unreliable transportation, taking the child to West Regional should have, at least, been considered. Had the base hospital agreed that the child's condition merited transportation to the closest facility, her wishes would have been met. If the child's condition worsened during transport to the more distant Central Children's Hospital and resulted in additional harm, up to and including death, the paramedic and the city he worked for would probably be sued.

The rank of a supervisor and the certification and training level of those who are supervised often conflict. An EMT may very well be the supervisor of a person holding an advanced life support (ALS) certification. On the EMS scene, an EMT supervisor can be required to defer to an ALS subordinate. This often creates conflicts that are difficult to manage and resolve. It is important to recognize that although the medical decisions of the paramedic supersede those of the EMT, the duties and responsibilities of a captain, such as managing potential agency liability, supersede those of the firefighter. The possibility of conflict and the potential types of conflict should be discussed prior to being placed in actual situations.

In this case study, the captain/EMT deferred, against her better judgment, allowing the patient to be transported to a hospital other than the closest appropriate facility. However, the supervisor chose to take appropriate action and discuss the incident with the paramedic charged with making that decision. She handled the situation quite well waiting for an appropriate time and place to speak with the paramedic. Additionally, she chose her words carefully, qualifying and validating the employee and using "I" statements rather than the accusatory "you" statements.

Hopefully, by discussing the potential ramifications, including patient outcomes, breaching of EMS protocols, as well as personal and agency liability, this type of conflict could be avoided in the future. It is imperative that all members of an EMS team communicate openly, honestly, and frequently, all directed toward improving patient care.

Lessons Learned

What Do You Know?

Engine 11 and Ambulance 14 were dispatched to an ill infant. Engine 11 was the first to arrive in the parking lot of a convenience store. They were met by the mother who was holding her infant daughter. After assessing the infant, the paramedic determined that she should be transported to the hospital. The mother consented but requested to go to West Regional Hospital because it was closer to her home and her car was not very reliable. The medic suggested that the infant be transported further away to Central Children's Hospital because of that hospital's pediatric specialization. The captain discussed this with the paramedic and discovered that the medic was biased against West Regional Hospital because he believed that they provided a lower standard of care. In the end, the infant was transported to Central Children's Hospital.

What Do You Need to Know?

EMS providers must be aware of the transport protocols of their system. EMS providers must also be aware of the chain of command and how the incident command system works in their system.

Resources

The medic in this case should have contacted the base hospital and obtained permission for the longer transport. If the infant was truly in need of a specialty hospital, it may be wise to consider the use of air transport. In this case, the engine crew may have wanted to inquire about public transportation or taxi cab vouchers that may have assisted the mother with her transportation needs.

Responsibilities

Every EMS provider has the responsibility to follow the transport protocols that exist in their system. If there is a need to deviate from these protocols, it should be done in consultation with a physician at the base hospital. EMS professionals also have the responsibility to follow the chain of command and work within the incident command system. Company officers and command officers have the responsibility to follow the treatment decisions of the EMS professional providing treatment. EMS professionals have the ethical responsibility to not let their personal biases interfere with treatment decisions.

Action Plan

In this case, the correct decision would have been to transport the infant to West Regional Hospital.

Justification of Your Action Plan

The infant should have been transported to West Regional Hospital as it was the closest facility that was able to provide the next level of care for this patient. Moreover, the mother of the patient requested transport to West Regional Hospital. EMS professionals should always respect the rights of patients and/or parents to select the hospital. The only time it is appropriate to override these wishes is in the case of a life-threatening condition.

Follow-up

In this case, it was appropriate for the captain to follow-up with the paramedic. Both the captain and the paramedic should take steps to ensure that personal biases do not interfere with treatment decisions in the future.

Summary

This case illustrates the difficulty that can arise when the chain of command and the issue of medical control are in conflict. EMS professionals can avoid these situations by discussing each other's expectations and being clear what is expected at each and every emergency scene. Although the captain did not have medical control at this scene, she is responsible for the overall incident. Because this crew did not listen to the mother's request to be transported to West Regional Hospital, it is possible that she may call to file a complaint. It is the captain's responsibility to see that the best customer service is provided on every call. It is also the captain's responsibility to see that standard operating procedures are followed.

The paramedic is likewise responsible to see that the best customer service is provided. As the senior EMS professional, the paramedic must ensure that the standard treatment and transport protocols are followed. By allowing his personal bias to influence his decision, he placed his captain and the rest of his crew at risk for a complaint. This is as much a supervision issue as it is a teamwork issue.

Key Terms

Biases   A personal and sometimes unreasoned prejudice in a general or specific sense, usually in the sense for having a preference to one particular person, place, thing, or idea.

Chain of Command   The line of authority and responsibility along which orders and directives are passed within an emergency response agency.

Incident Command System   A structured incident management system that is commonly employed at incidents in which span-of-control is an issue. The presence of an incident commander allows those treating the patients to focus on the task level, whereas the incident commander directs attention to strategy, safety, and resource management issues such as hospital and patient transportation availability.

Medical Control   Decisions regarding patient treatment and transport are the responsibility of the highest level EMS professional (paramedic, EMT, etc.) providing care to a specific patient. Medical control functions independently of the EMS professional's rank in the chain of command.

Transport Protocols   Every EMS system is required to develop and implement procedures governing the assessment and transportation of patients.

10

Bright Idea

Psychosocial, Ethical, and Leadership Dimensions

- Interagency Cooperation
- Mental Illness
- Safety

Bright Idea

Mark and Willie were sipping coffee at the White Fox Den. It was just past midnight and they still had a long way to go until their shift ended. They were both working on their second cup when they heard the dispatcher on their portable radio. "Rescue 5, ill person. See the sheriff. Barkley Lake picnic area off of State Route 47." They left a couple of dollars on the table, bundled up, and went outside where their ambulance was parked. It was cold outside and they could both see their breath. The wind was blowing in from the north and it stung their cheeks. Willie started the ambulance and Mark picked up the microphone. "Rescue 5 responding," he said.

It took about 12 minutes to get to Barkley Lake. As they approached the picnic area, they could see by the emergency lights that four patrol cars were parked at the far end. They pulled in and were met by Deputy Devin Brown. The three of them had all gone to high school together. Devin smiled as he saw who was in the ambulance. "Hi Willie. Hey Mark. Thanks for coming."

"Sure Devin, what's up?" inquired Willie.

"It's Brian Hall. We got called out because some folks spotted a campfire and the picnic area closes at ten. Thought we had some illegal campers. Turns out it was Brian. Poor kid is a mess. He thinks he is back in Iraq. We keep trying to talk with him but he thinks we're the insurgents. Threatens to shoot us if we get any closer, but as far as we can tell he's not armed. He keeps yelling out 'Bravo Four come in.' Sandy England's been trying to talk to him, but she ain't havin' much success."

"I remember Brian," said Mark. "He used to play football with my son Tommy."

"Yeah, that's him," acknowledged Devin. "Zack Greene is over talking to his folks. I guess he just hasn't been the same since he came back from the war."

"How can we help?" asked Willie.

"Well we thought we should get him over to the hospital so that Doc Griffin can take a look at him. We just don't know how to get him there. Like I said we've been trying to talk him down, and we don't want to take him down unless we absolutely have to. We think that will just make it worse for him. You guys got any ideas?" Devin looked at both of them hopefully.

Problem Solving

What Do You Know?

- Describe what you know about this incident.

What Do You Need to Know?

- What additional information would be helpful before further decision making?

Resources

- What potential resources would be helpful at this stage?

Responsibilities

- What legal, ethical, organizational, or interpersonal responsibilities should you consider?

Action Plan

- Decide what you would do next if you were in this situation.

Justification of Your Action Plan

- Explain the rationale you used for your decision.

Follow-up

- Would your action plan require any follow-up? Why or why not?

The Rest of the Story

Willie and Mark looked at each other not sure what to do. "You know him," Willie said to Mark.

"He used to play on the football team with my son. I didn't say I knew him real well," replied Mark.

"Could be a place to start," Willie suggested.

"Sandy's been talking to him for a while now," said Devin. "I don't think he knows who any of us are." There was a long silence. Everyone was deep in thought. They all wanted to help Brian. Finally, Mark spoke up.

"I have an idea. We'll need help from all your people too Devin."

"You got it," replied Devin enthusiastically.

Mark shared his plan. Devin nodded in agreement. He radioed the rest of the sheriff's deputies and briefed them on the plan. Willie pulled the ambulance forward, shut off the lights, and slowly backed toward the spot where Brian was hunkered down. He turned the ambulance off and waited. Sandy pulled back from her position, went over to her patrol car, shut off all the lights, and turned her car off. One by one, all the sheriff's deputies did the same thing. Suddenly, it was silent. The only light was from the moon and Brian's campfire. Everyone waited. After a time, the silence was broken by Brian's call, "Bravo Four, come in Bravo Four."

Mark picked up the microphone and turned on the ambulance's loudspeaker. "This is Bravo Four. Condition green; all clear. All units come on in." At the same time, Willie turned on the spotlight mounted on the back of the ambulance and threw the back door open. Brian looked up from his position and ran into the back of the ambulance. Mark met him and said, "Good job soldier. The insurgency has been turned away."

"Thank you sir," was Brian's reply.

Mark continued, "Soldier, I need you to let this medic check you out, make sure you weren't hit."

"Yes sir," Brian complied.

"Sit here," Mark instructed as he pointed to the gurney. "Medic Thompson is going to examine you while you tell me what happened out there."

"Yes sir."

"We're going to head back to base in this transport."

Devin climbed into the ambulance and drove them all to the hospital. Willie conducted an assessment and concluded that Brian was not injured. He and Mark listened intently while Brian told them a story about what had happened to him in Iraq.

Discussion

- What do you think of Mark and Willie's intervention?
- What could have gone wrong with this intervention?
- Do you think they violated any policies and procedures or EMS protocols?
- Was it appropriate for the sheriff's deputy to drive the ambulance to the hospital?
- Where do you transport patients like Brian in your jurisdiction?

Skill Building

This is an excellent example of interagency cooperation between local law enforcement and emergency medical service (EMS). The sheriff's deputies recognized that the use of force in this situation had the potential to escalate into violence. The use of force with EMS patients should be limited to situations where they present an immediate danger to themselves or others.

Brian, the patient in this case, was displaying symptoms of posttraumatic stress disorder (PTSD). PTSD is a type of anxiety disorder that emerges after an individual has experienced an extremely distressing event such as disaster, accident, physical or sexual assault, or combat. It is common for the individual to reexperience the event through dreams, recurrent thoughts, or images. Depending on the severity and the duration of the event, the individual can experience a detachment from the world, even to the point of psychosis. This was clearly the case with Brian. The signs and symptoms of PTSD also include hypervigilance, exaggerated startle response, heart palpitations, sleep disturbances, and gastrointestinal disturbances. Substance abuse can also be present as patients try to self-medicate. PTSD symptoms can be exacerbated by stress (Thomas & Woodall, 2006).

Mark and Willie demonstrated how a little creativity can help to reduce a patient's anxiety and help to gain control of a situation. Had they chosen to confront Brian's belief that he was still in Iraq, it is likely that he would have further decompensated and the standoff could have been quite lengthy. Furthermore, it could have escalated into a violent situation in the back of the ambulance. Some may criticize this approach as reinforcing Brian's delusional thinking. However, it is not the role of EMS responders to challenge and correct a patient's psychotic thinking. Brian needs to be treated with medications and therapy by licensed mental health professionals. It is possible that Brian could have been armed. Although the sheriff's deputy stated that "as far as we can tell he's not armed," Mark and Willie did put themselves at risk.

It is hard to know if Mark and Willie violated any of their agency's policies and procedures or EMS protocols. We would hope that they contacted their base hospital and gave an on-scene report regarding Brian's condition. It might have also been appropriate for them to contact the base hospital and/or a supervisor before proceeding with this type of intervention. Having the sheriff's deputy drive the ambulance may or may not be a violation of policy. In some communities, this may be the norm, particularly in rural areas where there are fewer resources. In any case, it also may have been prudent for them to notify their dispatcher or supervisor that this was taking place.

Lessons Learned

What Do You Know?

Rescue 5 provides EMS in a small community where most of the residents know each other. They are dispatched late one night to assist an ill person at a picnic area, a short way out of town. Rescue 5 arrives and meets a group of sheriff's deputies whom they are familiar with. The sheriff's deputies have been communicating with Brian, a young man from the town who is known to all of them. Brian is a soldier who recently returned from Iraq and is suffering from PTSD. Brian appears to be delusional and has been calling out for "Bravo Four," behaving as if he is back in Iraq. The deputies have determined that Brian is unarmed and have been negotiating with him for some time, trying to get him to the hospital for an evaluation. Having little success, they contacted EMS for assistance.

One of the EMS providers develops a plan to get Brian into the ambulance. They moved the ambulance into the scene and shut it down. They made all the deputies shut down their patrol cars until the area is quiet. When Brian calls out for Bravo Four, one of the EMS professionals responds as if he is Bravo Four and gives the "all clear" command. He requests Brian to come in and report. Brian climbs into the ambulance and is examined. The EMS providers remain in the back of the ambulance with him while one of the deputies drives them to the hospital.

What Do You Need to Know?

EMS professionals should have knowledge of any policies and procedures regarding interagency cooperation. EMS professionals routinely interact with law enforcement, fire departments, and other EMS agencies. EMS professionals may also have cause to work with public utilities, volunteer agencies, and private contractors.

Resources

It is a good practice for emergency responders to be aware of any services that are available to veterans in their area. This may include a hospital, clinic, and rehabilitation facilities. In some cases, patients may request transport to a Veterans Administration (VA) hospital because they can receive care there at no cost. Emergency responders should always try to honor a patient's request to be transported to a VA hospital.

Responsibilities

Emergency responders have the responsibility to maintain their personal safety and the safety of the crew members. It could be said that this same level of responsibility should be extended in maintaining the personal safety of every emergency responder at the scene. EMS professionals also have the responsibility to make sure that the safety of their patients and the public is always maintained.

In this case, Mark and Willie took the deputy's word that Brian was not armed. That does not lessen the fact that they put themselves in potential danger by allowing Brian to enter the ambulance without first being searched and cleared by the sheriff's deputies. This step is important for ensuring their safety, the deputies' safety, and Brian's safety.

Action Plan

In most cases, it is law enforcement's responsibility to secure patients who are barricaded or are being uncooperative. EMS professionals are not trained in restraint techniques and should not place themselves in situations where they could be harmed. Although the outcome of this intervention was successful, the potential for something to go wrong was very high.

Justification of Your Action Plan

EMS providers should always wait until a scene has been secured before treating a patient. It is not the responsibility of EMS providers to negotiate and resolve barricade or hostage situations.

Follow-up

Given that this is a small community, it might be appropriate for Mark and Willie to check with Brian and/or his family to see how he is doing. Events such as this have the potential to embarrass the patient and his or her family. Brian and his family may take some small comfort knowing that the EMS providers who treated him were compassionate and empathetic to his situation.

Summary

This case is a good example of interagency cooperation. Here the EMS crew worked in conjunction with the sheriff's office to successfully resolve a difficult situation calmly and peaceably. It is interesting to note that a sheriff's deputy drove the ambulance to the hospital. It begs the question of whether this is a common or excepted practice. Although it seemed like the logical and right thing to do, it may have opened the door to other potential risks. What if the ambulance had been involved in a crash on the way to the hospital? Someone would surely ask the question of whether the deputy was authorized to drive the ambulance. The wise thing would be to get permission from the on-duty supervisor of both agencies. Some could say that the small size and closeness of this community facilitated this cooperation. Even though that may be true, there have been many examples of interagency cooperation in large metropolitan areas.

The fact that this was a small community where everyone knows each other could also be seen as a contributing factor in the safety issue in this case. Sometimes when a patient is known to the emergency responders, it becomes all too easy to relax and feel comfortable with the patient. This can happen when the patient is a friend or relative of the EMS provider, or because the EMS provider has treated the patient on multiple occasions in the past. Just because we know someone does not mean that they are going to behave in the same way that they did in the past. Many medical and psychological conditions can result in altered behavior. EMS professionals should seek to maintain a high level of safety awareness in these situations.

Patients with mental illness are prone to have significant changes in the mood and behavior. This can be a result of changes in, or non-compliance with, prescription medication. In some psychological disorders, behavior changes are experienced as one of the symptoms of the disorder. EMS professionals should also be aware that substance abuse may cause significant changes in a person's behavior.

Key Terms

Anxiety   A vague, unpleasant emotional state with the qualities of apprehension, dread, distress, and uneasiness.

Decompensate   A term that describes the increasing severity of psychological symptoms accompanied by deterioration in mental and social functioning.

Delusion   A belief that is maintained in spite of argument, data, and refutation that should (reasonably) be sufficient to destroy it.

Detachment   The lack of feeling or emotional involvement in a problem, situation, or interactions with another person.

Empathetic   A cognitive awareness and understanding of the emotions and feelings of another person.

Exaggerated Startle Response   A complex reaction to a sudden, unanticipated stimulus. The stimulus may be real or imagined. There is flexion of most skeletal muscles and various visceral and hormonal reactions.

Hypervigilance   State of being associated with extreme carefulness, awareness to the possibility of danger or injury.

Interagency Cooperation   The collaboration of more than one agency to meet a specified objective.

Post-traumatic Stress Disorder   A type of anxiety disorder that emerges after a psychologically distressing traumatic event such as disaster, accident, war, and rape.

Psychosis   Often used to describe a set of symptoms characterized by delusional thinking and/or hallucinations.

Psychotic Condition   Referring to the total mental condition of a person who has suffered a break from reality at a specific moment.

References

Thomas, J., & Woodall, S. J. (2006). *Responding to Psychological Emergencies: A Field Guide.* Clifton Park, NY: Thomson-Delmar Learning.

11

One Patient— To Go

Psychosocial, Ethical, and Leadership Dimensions

- Customer Service
- Patient Advocacy
- Team Dynamics
- EMS Protocols
- Health and Wellness
- Standard Operating Procedures

One Patient—To Go

It was almost 11 pm when Ambulance 202 left the emergency bay at Northwest Receiving Hospital. They had just transported a 6-year-old boy having a severe asthma attack. The paramedics were both tired. They had been on the go since the beginning of their shift. The weather outside was hot and sticky. They hadn't been driving for more than a minute when they were dispatched to assist Engine 101 with a fall injury. They both breathed a heavy sigh as they kicked on the lights and siren. Instinctively, they both knew they were in for a long night.

Because of the weather, the entire EMS system was on overload. The fire and EMS crews were running all over the town on heat-related emergencies. As a result of the overload, they were traveling far out of their usual response area and it would take almost 10 minutes to get to the location of the fall injury. They were headed to lower downtown near the rail yards. Heavy traffic leaving the baseball stadium slowed their response even more. As they responded, the medics wondered who had won the game. Laboring through the traffic, they finally arrived on the scene. The response had taken a full 14 minutes.

To their surprise, Engine 101 was nowhere in sight. What they found surprised them even more. There on the street was an adult male strapped to a backboard. His head was blocked, with a C-collar around his neck, and an EMS form was tucked in next to his right ear. Having never encountered anything like this before, neither one of them was quite sure what to do. They checked the computer in the ambulance and it showed that Engine 101 was still on the scene.

Problem Solving

What Do You Know?

- Describe what you know about this incident.

What Do You Need to Know?

- What additional information would be helpful before further decision making?

Resources

- What potential resources would be helpful at this stage?

Responsibilities

- What legal, ethical, organizational, or interpersonal responsibilities should you consider?

Action Plan

- Decide what you would do next if you were in this situation.

Justification of Your Action Plan

- Explain the rationale you used for your decision.

Follow-up

- Would your action plan require any follow-up? Why or why not?

The Rest of the Story

Still not sure what to do, the two medics reassessed the patient. They found him to be slightly intoxicated but otherwise stable. Based on his clothing, they surmised that the man was probably homeless. The EMS form indicated that the patient was to be transported to Downtown General. Not wanting to cause any problem with the engine company and not wanting to fill out any extra paperwork, the two medics loaded the patient into the ambulance and transported him to Downtown General.

Discussion

- Did the Engine 101 crew violate any standard emergency medical service (EMS) protocols?
- Did the Ambulance 202 medics violate any standard EMS protocols?

- Did the Ambulance 202 medics violate any agency protocols or standard operating procedures (SOPs)?
- Did the Engine 101 crew expose themselves and their agency to any potential liability?
- Did the Ambulance 202 medics expose themselves and their agency to any potential liability?
- Suggest some other strategies that the Ambulance 202 medics could have used in this situation.
- Do you think that a homeless patient receives a different standard of care than is usually provided to the general public? Why or why not?

Skill Building

Several factors contribute to a situation like this. Clearly, there are some things going on with the Engine 101 crew. The actions on the part of Ambulance 202 suggest that there may be larger problems in the agency as a whole. This case also speaks to the problem of homelessness and other people who are marginalized from mainstream society.

After running countless EMS calls, there will be times when our patience runs thin. Sometimes our anger and frustration is because we are hungry, tired, and feel overworked. Sometimes it is because we want to hurry up and get out of the weather. Sometimes it is because we are in need of some time off. Sometimes it is because we are experiencing problems in our personal lives. Sadly enough, sometimes it is because we are experiencing a case of compassion fatigue or burnout. It is important for each of us to monitor ourselves for the signs of compassion fatigue. Pfifferling and Gilley (2000) defined compassion fatigue with the following set of symptoms:

- Lack of motivation
- Poor performance
- Making excuses for poor performance

- Belittling and offensive labels for customers
- Dark humor
- Overconfidence
- Disregard for standard EMS protocols
- Violations of agency operating guidelines
- Chronic complaining
- Irritability
- Patient abuse
- Creating bureaucracy
- Missing work
- Social withdrawal
- Drug or alcohol abuse

If you find yourself experiencing several of these symptoms, remember that compassion fatigue is common among emergency responders. It is important, however, that you recognize that something needs to be done. The solution could be as simple as taking a few shifts off, or it could be that it is time to talk with someone you trust or even to a mental health professional. Many EMS agencies have critical incident stress management programs in place. Many employers offer employee assistance programs (EAPs) that will allow you to talk with a professional at little or no charge.

It is easy to speculate about what was going on with the Engine 101 crew. One thing is for certain: there was a critical breakdown in supervision within this crew. In order for a patient to be left unattended, the supervisor, in this case the captain, had to be complicit in the act. It is the captain's responsibility to lead by example and to make sure that incidents such as this do not happen. Often supervisors make the mistake of wanting to become "one of the crew." In doing so, they may forgo their supervisory responsibilities. What starts out as a little joke can lead to tragic consequences for the patient, the crew, and your career. The captain or the supervisor sets the tone for the entire crew. If the supervisor is suffering from burnout, the bad attitude will be contagious and soon the crew will be affected. The paramedics on this engine are also guilty of abandoning this patient. They have placed their hard-earned professional certifications in jeopardy if someone was to report their actions.

The Ambulance 202 crew was also a part of the problem. Though they did a thorough assessment of the patient, they chose not to report Engine 101's actions. That choice made them accomplices in the patient abuse and patient abandonment. The rationale for doing this could be the result of their own burnout, or it could be indicative of some organizational problems. They could have reported to the person who was responsible to the hospital or to their immediate supervisor how they found this patient. At the very minimum, a discussion should have taken place with Engine 101 about the incident and a warning given that it would be reported if it was to happen again. Please be advised that addressing this incident at the crew level would fall far short of what your supervising agency would want or expect.

If an agency is experiencing a high rate of compassion fatigue among its members, it may not be doing the best job that it could. Some factors to consider are: Is the agency fully staffed? Is the call volume such that additional response units are needed? Could it be the result of not doing enough for the members in the area of health and wellness? The ambulance crew not wanting to cause problems with the engine company hints that a dysfunctional dynamic may exist between the ambulance crews and the engine companies. The paperwork excuse may be indicative of bureaucratic impediments that prevent employees from doing the right thing.

Another factor may be the fact that this man appeared to be homeless. This illustrates the fact that marginalized people are often the ones who are mistreated. There is a false belief that these people will not report the mistreatment because they are solely dependent on the system to take care of their needs. Perhaps they felt that because he was intoxicated, he would not remember what had happened to him. Whatever the case, the Engine 101 crew concluded that it was in some way OK for them to mistreat, neglect, and abandon this man and Ambulance 202 enabled their behavior.

The homeless rely on social services more than any other portion of the population. They have no resources or anyone to call. Often they are mentally ill or addicted to drugs or alcohol. They depend on the good graces of society to assist them.

Our mission is to serve as advocates for all we serve, no matter what their social status or perceived or real condition. We must never lose sight of our mission and our responsibility to self-police and monitor our progress.

Lessons Learned

What Do You Know?

The Engine 101 crew treated and stabilized a patient and left him strapped to a backboard, outdoors, during a heat wave. An ambulance had been called to transport the patient, but it is unknown how long the patient had been abandoned as the ambulance computer indicated that Engine 101 was still on the scene. The ambulance crew reassessed the patient and found him to be intoxicated but otherwise stable. The patient's clothing indicated that he was probably homeless. Following the instructions of the Engine 101 crew, they transported the patient to the hospital.

What Do You Need to Know?

Not that it matters, but it would be helpful to know just what motivated Engine 101 to abandon this patient. Most certainly, they were not following EMS protocols and department's SOPs. More information regarding the track record of this crew could shed more light on this situation. Finally, understanding what could possibly have motivated these individuals to collectively exercise such poor judgment.

Resources

Before making a decision to abandon a patient, all other potential resources must be exhaustively examined. A taxi cab could be a resource, and although it would constitute breaking a common SOP, the crew could have even considered loading the patient on the hose bed along with one or two firefighters to secure him and driven very slowly to the closest hospital. Another resource option would be to call the shift supervisor for advice and assistance. The shift supervisor may have been able to transport the patient if his or her rig was capable of accommodating a patient strapped to a backboard.

Responsibilities

The Engine 101 supervisor should have made a command decision to stay with the patient until the ambulance arrived to transport him to the hospital. Legally, this crew could be held responsible if this patient suffered further injury or death due in any part to the condition in which they left him. Patient abandonment also constitutes a serious breach of Advanced Life Support (ALS) and Basic Life Support (BLS) medical protocol. If the Engine 101 crew were found guilty of breaching this medical protocol, they would most likely lose their certification as EMS providers. Upon arrival, Ambulance 202 should have called for a supervisor.

When examining this scenario from the organizational and interpersonal responsibility perspective, it is obvious that the Engine 101 crew's actions would only discredit their agency, the fire/EMS community, and their individual professional reputations. Moreover, what do their actions say to the public at large and other social agencies that serve the underprivileged and homeless?

Action Plan

The best and most viable action plan would be to stay with this patient until the ambulance arrived to transport him to the hospital. We are called to one emergency at a time and must commit ourselves to completely and thoroughly meeting that patient's needs before moving on to the next emergency. Again, it must be emphasized that Ambulance 202 should have contacted Engine 101 when they were on the scene and then contacted the shift supervisor.

Justification of Your Action Plan

A plan that is formulated in sound, professional judgment, designed to produce a positive and desirable outcome, and is in the best interest of the patient will not need any justification. Engine 101's actions did not demonstrate any of the components of a well-thought-out, well-executed plan. Furthermore, the Ambulance 202 crew's decision not to report this incident could be considered an enabling behavior that would only encourage Engine 101 to act irresponsibly and unethically in the future. Risk management is the responsibility of every member of the agency. This agency was facing the possibility of litigation and the responding personnel were facing the possibility of losing their EMS certifications. Disciplinary action should be taken in this case.

Follow-up

Minimally, Ambulance 202 should absolutely follow-up with Engine 101. Justification of Engine 101's actions should most definitely be discussed. All parties would need to assure each other that this would never happen again.

Ethically, organizationally, and morally, Ambulance 202 should document the incident and forward the report up the chain of command. This effort would be taken with the hope of minimizing the chances of this type of patient care happening in the future. And finally, getting back to the mission, someone should be tasked with patient follow-up. A phone call or visit should be made to the Downtown General Emergency Department to check on the welfare of the abused patient and to make sure that the proper social services agencies were notified of this man's homeless situation.

Summary

Action plans should always incorporate strategies that work within the law, agency SOPs, EMS protocols, and most importantly common sense. We should also always be cognizant of our role as patient advocates, paying special attention to our patients' right to human dignity and respect and never treating anyone as a lesser being. Finally, we should adhere to customer service guidelines and use the positive aspects of team dynamics to exercise peer pressure to do things right and do the right things.

The desire to cover for the mistakes of our fellow employees can be quite a dilemma. The public greatly frowns on perceived or real cover-ups that only serve to make matters worse rather than better. If this patient had died or the actions of these crews led to a less than desirable outcome, the actions of these EMS crews would be considered criminal.

Key Terms

Compassion Fatigue   Commonly referred to as "burnout," this term describes individuals usually working in the helping professions who have, for various reasons, lost their ability to effectively manage their personal and professional relationships with work team members, family members, supervisors, and those they serve. This is frequently caused by overwork, continual exposure to the negative aspects of the human condition, and fatigue including sleep deprivation.

Employee Assistance Program   A benefit program provided by the employer who usually offers assessment, short-term counseling, and referral services.

EMS Protocols   Guidelines for prehospital patient care.

Enabling Behavior   Behaviors and actions that allow others to continue dysfunctional, unethical, illegal, or harmful behavior(s).

Homelessness   Intentionally or unintentionally being without a permanent home that would provide for what is considered normal amenities such as a bed, shower, kitchen, and restroom.

Patient Abandonment   The discontinuation of medical treatment at a time when continuing care would normally be required.

Standard Operating Procedure   A written set of procedures that define a particular task to be performed in a step-by-step format.

References

Pfifferling, J. H., & Gilley, K. (2000). Overcoming Compassion Fatigue. *Family Practice Management* 7(4).

12

Pain in the Butt

Psychosocial, Ethical, and Leadership Dimensions

- Customer Service
- Patient Advocacy
- Teamwork
- Unconditional Positive Regard

Pain in the Butt

It was a beautiful morning and the crew had just finished doing their truck check. Everything was in working order and there were no problems to report. The crew had just settled into the watch room to check their e-mail and catch up on paperwork when, the first call came, "abdominal pain." The crew jumped on the fire engine and headed off to a residence in an upper-middle-class suburb. While responding Code 3, they were able to ascertain that the patient was a 42-year-old male.

When they arrived at the home, they grabbed their EMS gear and proceeded to the front door. One of the firefighter EMTs rang the bell and waited for someone to answer. No response. The crew rang a couple more times and then tried the door. The door was unlocked, so the EMT opened it slightly and in a loud voice said, "Fire department!"

"I'm in here" was the reply that came from the master bedroom in the back of the house. As soon as the crew walked in, they knew something was terribly wrong. The stench that greeted them was overwhelming. It smelled like a sewer had exploded inside the house. Carefully making their way to the master bedroom, they noticed dark spots on the carpet. The odor was strong, but nothing could have prepared them for what they encountered. There on the bed was a grown man lying in a vast amount of his own feces.

"Thank God you're here!" exclaimed the man. "I am really sick and I can't stop it!" Not sure what to do first, the captain/paramedic asked the man how long this has been going on. "Days," came the reply. "See that on the wall? It just keeps shooting out of me!"

This was easy for the crew to believe as they just stood there, still somewhat bewildered by the scene in front of them. "We're going to check you out," the captain/paramedic told him. By this time, the crew had begun to don protective sleeves, gowns, and HEPA masks. The crew did the best they could to clean up the man and do a basic assessment. His vital signs were normal and he only had a slight temperature. His abdomen was soft, but he complained of pain and discomfort when it was palpated. As they were finishing the assessment, the man exclaimed, "Look out, I gotta go again!"

At this point, the second paramedic barked at the man, "Get out of bed and get on the toilet!" Without missing a beat, the two EMTs pulled the man off the bed and sat him on the toilet.

Problem Solving

What Do You Know?

- Describe what you know about this incident.

What Do You Need to Know?

- What additional information would be helpful before further decision making?

Resources

- What potential resources would be helpful at this stage?

Responsibilities

- What legal, ethical, organizational, or interpersonal responsibilities should you consider?

Action Plan

- Decide what you would do next if you were in this situation.

Justification of Your Action Plan

- Explain the rationale you used for your decision.

Follow-up

- Would your action require any follow-up? Why or why not?

The Rest of the Story

The ambulance crew arrived as the man was sitting on the toilet. The captain/paramedic radioed the hospital and advised them to expect a patient suffering from explosive diarrhea. "The ambulance is here and we are going to take you to the hospital," he informed the man.

"I can't go anywhere like this!" exclaimed the man from his seat on the toilet. The second paramedic told the man, "Get up and get into the shower or we are taking you in just like this." One of the EMTs helped the man into the shower, so he could clean himself up. The captain/paramedic retrieved some clean clothes and allowed him to dress before sitting on the gurney. They started an IV and transported him to the hospital where he was treated for an intestinal virus.

Discussion

- Did this crew provide the best possible service?
- What did they do right in this situation?
- Did they do anything wrong?
- How will you react when confronted by a patient like this?

Skill Building

This is a good example of great customer service. Often times EMS responders see people at their worst. It is important to remember that one of the best treatments we can offer is helping people to reclaim their dignity. Although it would have been easy to quickly load this patient and transport him to the hospital, this crew took the extra time to allow the man to shower and dress. There are various reasons why patients are unable to attend to or choose not to take care of their hygiene. It may be the result of a medical condition that leaves them physically unable to wash; patients with mental illness are sometimes unaware that they have neglected their hygiene; physical disabilities, developmental disabilities, and morbid obesity can sometimes make it difficult for individuals to clean themselves. Substance abuse can also play a role in poor hygiene. Some might argue that taking extra time to help patients clean themselves, or cleaning the patients yourselves, delays transport and lengthens the amount of time that EMS units spend on a call. No matter what the cause, EMS responders need to be aware that these patients are vulnerable and often embarrassed by their condition. This case is also an example of the need to expect the unexpected. This type of patient encounter was probably not something they expected at the start of their shift. To their credit, this crew also took all the proper body substance isolation (BSI) precautions. By taking the time to don full personal protective equipment (PPE), they reduced their risk of exposure (Thomas & Woodall, 2006). Using PPE also allowed them to more fully engage this patient and do a thorough assessment. By cleaning up this patient and allowing him to shower and dress, they also demonstrated consideration for the ambulance crew and the hospital staff who would be transporting and treating this patient, respectively.

Lastly, this crew exhibited what is known as unconditional positive regard. This philosophy of care espouses that all patients be treated with respect, dignity, and compassion regardless of their condition, circumstances, or personal characteristics. Patients who are treated with unconditional positive regard experience positive interactions with healthcare providers, respond better to treatment, and recover more rapidly (Rogers, 1951; Sheldon, 2004).

Lessons Learned

What Do You Know?

The engine crew was dispatched to respond to a 42-year-old man with abdominal pain. When they arrived at his residence, they discovered the man lying in bed covered with his own feces. The man indicated that he had been experiencing uncontrollable diarrhea for the past few days. As they were assessing him, the man reported that he was about to lose control of his bowels again. The crew placed the man on the toilet and informed him that he would need to go to the hospital. Before transporting him, the crew assisted him in taking a shower and putting on clean clothes. He was transported to the hospital and treated for an intestinal virus.

What Do You Need to Know?

EMS professionals need to be aware of and follow BSI precautions. Body substances can pose a hazard to first responders. Communicable diseases such as hepatitis B and C, HIV, meningitis, pneumonia, mumps, tuberculosis, chicken pox, staph infection, and pertussis can be spread to individuals who do not properly protect themselves from exposure. The Centers for Disease Control (1989) and the National Fire Protection Association (2007) recommend that all first responders and healthcare providers use PPE. EMS providers should also be aware that a patient who has lost a great deal of bodily fluids may be severely dehydrated.

Resources

From this story, it is unclear why this man was not able to get himself to the toilet and was unable or unwilling to attend to his personal hygiene. His behavior could be the result of something more than just an intestinal virus. In making their report at the hospital, the medics could have advised that the patient may benefit from a psychological evaluation.

Responsibilities

Emergency responders have the obligation to help patients preserve their dignity and modesty whenever possible. Providers also have the responsibility to be considerate of other professionals in the EMS system. Some crews may have decided to wrap this patient in a sheet and transport as quickly as possible. Cleaning up this patient would then have become the responsibility of another EMS provider. Transporting as quickly as possible would show disregard for the patient's dignity and little consideration for the staff at the hospital.

Action Plan

If a patient is able to clean himself of herself, the EMS crew should allow a patient the time to clean up. If a patient is unable to clean himself of herself, the EMS crew should, at the very least, wipe off the patient with a towel. This is not a pleasant task, but it is necessary to do a good visual assessment. In addition, the transport of bodily substances is a violation of standard BSI precautions.

Justification of Your Action Plan

Cleaning up the patient is mandated by EMS protocols and BSI precautions.

Follow-up

If treating this patient resulted in the exposure of an EMS provider to bodily substances, it must be reported to the agency's safety officer. It might also be wise to check with the hospital regarding the diagnosis. This could be especially important in the case of an exposure.

Summary

This case is a good example of effective teamwork and good leadership. No doubt the crew was uncomfortable in this situation. The fact that the paramedic "barked" at the man indicates just how high the tension must have been. During the entire call, the captain remained calm and even retrieved clean clothes for the man. By remaining calm and not allowing himself to get caught up in the crew's tension, the captain ensured the best possible outcome for this patient.

The captain also provided a great example of unconditional positive regard. He treated the man with respect and dignity; he also did not rush to any judgments. EMS professionals must be mindful of the fact that we frequently see people when they are most vulnerable. The potential for embarrassment is great. What we don't know when we arrive on scene is what transpired that would allow for someone to engage in this type of behavior. It is easy to lose sight of the fact that a number of precipitating factors may have contributed to this situation.

Even though they were uncomfortable, the crew displayed exceptional customer service in this case. Had they acted on their frustration and discomfort, they may have treated this patient poorly. Poor service can often result in a citizen complaint. In his book *Essentials of Fire Department Customer Service*, Alan Brunacini (1996) stated that people do not always remember the particular examinations or medical treatments that were administered, but what they do remember is how they were treated.

Finally, this crew showed great respect for the other providers in the EMS system. They chose not to pass an unpleasant state of affairs along to the hospital. They recognized that the patient's condition could potentially have a negative impact on his treatment at the hospital. They also chose to take proper BSI precautions and not to contaminate the emergency department. Had they chosen not to take the actions they did, it may have damaged their standing and relationship with the hospital staff.

Key Terms

BSI   It describes the actions taken by the EMS provider to ensure that those working with a patient are not unnecessarily exposed to the body substances emanating from a patient or patients.

Developmental Disabilities   Physical or mental conditions that show what is considered to be the normal psychological developmental process.

Morbid Obesity   The state of being overweight to the point that a person's normal life expectancy is greatly reduced.

PPE   For EMS calls, this equipment is composed of latex gloves, eye protection, substance resistance pull on sleeves, gowns, and filtering masks. In fire situations, PPE would consist of turnout gear, helmet, boots, and a self-contained breathing apparatus (SCBA).

Unconditional Positive Regard   Treating patients with respect and dignity and viewing them as worthy and capable, even when they do not act or feel that way.

References

Brunacini, A. V. (1996). *Essentials of Fire Department Customer Service.* Stillwater, OK: Fire Protection Publications.

Centers for Disease Control (1989). *Guidelines for Prevention of Transmission of Human Immunodeficiency Virus and Hepatitis B Virus to Health-Care and Public-Safety Workers A Response to P.L. 100-607 The Health Omnibus Programs Extension Act of 1988.* Atlanta, GA: Centers for Disease Control.

National Fire Protection Association (2007). *NFPA 1500: Standard on Fire Department Occupational Safety and Health Program*, 2007 edition. Quincy, MA: National Fire Protection Association.

Rogers, C. (1951). *Client-Centered Therapy: Its Current Practice, Implications and Theory.* London, UK: Constable.

Sheldon, L. (2004). *Communication for Nurses: Talking with Patients.* Boston, MA: Jones & Bartlett.

Thomas, J., & Woodall, S. J. (2006). *Responding to Psychological Emergencies: A Field Guide.* Clifton Park, NY: Thomson-Delmar Learning.

13

Fatal Mistake

Psychosocial, Ethical, and Leadership Dimensions

- Customer Service
- Death
- Grief
- Interagency Cooperation
- Interpersonal Skills

▓▓▓▓▓▓ Fatal Mistake

Hillman River prides itself on its volunteer fire department. The Hillman River Volunteer Fire Department operates out of one station. They provide fire protection, emergency medical service, and emergency transport for their small rural community. Advanced life support is available only by helicopter. The firehouse is a gathering point for the community. The volunteers host a community picnic in the summer and parents always take their children to see Santa at the annual Christmas Party. People in this small town take great comfort knowing that their neighbors are there to take care of them.

It was early in the morning when Wayne heard the siren. He was getting ready to go out and feed the animals; instead, he climbed into his truck and headed to the firehouse. Pete Collier was already sitting in the rescue squad when Wayne pulled up. He hopped into the passenger seat and buckled up his seat belt. He turned on the lights and siren as Pete pulled out of the garage. "What we got?" he asked Pete.

Pete had a troubled look on his face. "Possible suicide out at the Mulvaney's." "Bill Cowan's out there. He said that it was Kevin." In Hillman River, everyone knew everyone else. There were no strangers. Wayne instantly knew who Pete was talking about. Kevin Mulvaney was a 14-year-old boy who was a freshman in high school. He played on the basketball team, was active in the Boy Scouts, and liked to ride horses. Wayne found it hard to believe that Kevin would want to kill himself.

By the time they got to the Mulvaney's home, another police officer had arrived. It was Brad Hughes; he met them in the driveway. "It's Kevin!" Brad told them excitedly. "He's tried to hang himself. He's in his bedroom." Pete and Wayne grabbed the EMS equipment and followed Brad into the house. They passed through the living room. Officer Bill Cowan was doing his best to console the Mulvaneys. Brad Hughes led them back to the boy's bedroom. Pete and Wayne were both shocked by what they saw.

Kevin Mulvaney was naked and hanging lifeless on the bottom bunk of the bunk bed. He was on his knees and his upper body was supported by the necktie he had tied to the top bunk rail and then around his neck. A pornographic magazine was on the bed below his face. Pete and Wayne looked at each other in disbelief. They stood there for a second or two until Wayne reached out and placed his hand on Kevin's neck to feel for a pulse. Kevin's skin was cold, pale, and rubbery. There was no pulse. He felt for a pulse on his left arm and found that it was stiff. Wayne observed that blood had pooled in the bottom of his abdomen. He looked at Pete and Brad and just shook his head back and forth. Not one of them said a word.

Problem Solving

What Do You Know?

- Describe what you know about this incident.

What Do You Need to Know?

- What additional information would be helpful before further decision making?

Resources

- What potential resources would be helpful at this stage?

Responsibilities

- What legal, ethical, organizational, or interpersonal responsibilities should you consider?

Action Plan

- Decide what you would do next if you were in this situation.

Justification of Your Action Plan

- Explain the rationale you used for your decision.

Follow-up

- Would your action plan require any follow-up? Why or why not?

The Rest of the Story

"What are we going to say to his parents?" asked Pete.

"What can you say to someone when their son commits suicide?" Wayne lamented.

"I don't think it's a suicide fellas," Brad said shaking his head. "I read a report about this once. I think he was suffocating himself while he was masturbating."

"You may be right," agreed Pete. "I remember hearing something about a rock singer who died from it."

"You can't tell his parents that," pleaded Wayne. "No parent wants to hear that their son died while he was masturbating. Besides, we don't know for sure if that's what happened."

"He was looking at a porno mag," countered Pete.

"You can't tell them that," insisted Wayne. "It's bad enough they have lost their son. They don't want to remember him that way."

Brad put his hand up to stop the argument. "We'll let the coroner determine the cause of death," he said. "We can tell them we are sorry and that there was nothing we could do." "If they ask questions, I'm going to tell them what I think." Wayne and Pete nodded. Brad was the police officer and he was in charge of this scene. They exited the bedroom very carefully so as not to disturb any potential evidence. The three of them joined the others in the living room and did their best to comfort their grieving neighbors.

Discussion

- Is there anything else that Pete and Wayne could have done with Kevin?
- What would you tell Mr. and Mrs. Mulvaney if you were in this situation?
- What types of problems are encountered when treating a patient whom you know personally?

Skill Building

The process of intentionally reducing the amount of oxygen flowing to the brain while masturbating is known as autoerotic asphyxiation (AEA). The purpose of this behavior is to increase sexual pleasure and not self-destruction. Decreased oxygen flow is usually accomplished through self-strangulation or by placing a plastic bag over the head to induce suffocation. Most victims of AEA have attempted to rig some sort of fail-safe or self-rescue mechanism, such as a slipknot or hanging themselves from a height that would easily allow them to stand up. Death occurs when the victim becomes weak and disoriented from hypoxia and is unable to initiate the self-rescue mechanism.

Exact figures regarding the incidence of AEA are difficult to find. The practice of AEA occurs throughout the world and is found in every ethnic and socioeconomic group. Typically, the victims are adolescent or young adult males (Clark, 1996). Many emergency responders are unaware of what to look for and AEA deaths are often reported as intentional suicides. This is likely because of the fact that hanging is the second most common form of suicide by males in this age group (Baker et al., 1992). Additionally, many victims are found by their parents, who "clean up" the scene before emergency responders arrive. Current estimates place the incidence rate between 250 and 1000 deaths annually (Jenkins, 2000). Even though the potential for death is high, the practice of AEA should not be classified as a suicide. The intent of the behavior is clearly for sexual pleasure and death from AEA should be classified as accidental.

Suicide is a self-inflicted death in which the patient acts intentionally, directly, and consciously (Thomas & Woodall, 2006). Although Kevin's act put him at risk for death, it cannot be said that he acted in a conscious way to intentionally kill himself. Therefore, it would be erroneous to call his death a suicide. The correct term for this type of behavior is subintentional death. Subintentional death is a classification that refers to ill-defined deaths and practices that lead toward death.

Types of subintentional deaths among adolescents include drug abuse, risk taking when driving automobiles, and the careless handling of firearms (Comer, 2007).

In this case, Pete and Wayne did everything that they should have done with Kevin. The description of Kevin's body indicates that he had been deceased for some time. Because they were volunteer firefighters, they were not trained as paramedics and therefore were under no orders to contact a base hospital or use a cardiac monitor to verify death. They also resisted the temptation to cut the necktie and cover Kevin's body. Although this may seem like a caring thing to do, it is important to remember that this is a potential crime scene and the coroner will need to conduct an investigation. This will include taking photographs of the scene. It is important for emergency responders not to disturb any potential evidence in the scene where an investigation will take place. Once they determined that Kevin was deceased, control of this scene transferred to law enforcement.

Even though there was nothing to be done for Kevin, Pete and Wayne have a responsibility to provide survivor care for Mr. and Mrs. Mulvaney. The Mulvaneys are going through a very traumatic experience. It is quite possible that they may be displaying physical symptoms related to stress. Common reactions might include heart palpitations, tachycardia, hypertension, increased respiration, and/ or pressure in the chest (Thomas & Woodall, 2006). It would be appropriate for Pete and Wayne to take a set of vital signs on each of the parents. It is also important that they state that Kevin has died and express their condolences. Although this may seem like a formality, the definitive statement allows for the grieving process to begin.

Mr. and Mrs. Mulvaney should be told the truth about what happened to Kevin. Parents will have different reactions when being told that their child died from AEA as opposed to suicide. In both cases, parents are likely to experience a sense of shame and embarrassment. However, parents who survive a child's suicide must contend with guilt and self-blame. They may spend a long time questioning if they missed warning signs or should have done something differently. Saddling parents with this burden is unfair if the death was not truly a suicide. Although it may seem like a favor not to tell them that their son died from AEA, it is important to remember that this is the truth that they are going to find out in the future.

Survivor care includes telling the family what has happened in clear, concise, simple language. Relate the information in a calm, patient, and understanding manner. All questions should be answered tactfully and honestly. The role of the medical examiner should be explained, so that they can be prepared for what will happen next. EMS providers should avoid any judgments regarding the circumstances of the death. Survivors should never be left alone. Stay with them until someone else arrives. If need be, help them to contact family, friends, and/or clergy, so that they can begin to access their social support systems. Keep in mind that there are many different social, religious, cultural, and ethnic traditions with regard to how people react to death (Thomas & Woodall, 2006).

This case also presents the issue of responding to calls that involve family and friends. If at all possible, EMS responders should avoid treating family members. It is hard to remain objective and the provider will be experiencing his or her own grief reaction. It also removes the possibility of the provider working on a family member and having a less than favorable outcome. If need be, the responder can render care until another EMS provider arrives and takes over. There may be times when we may be called on to treat coworkers or someone we know socially. This is especially true in small communities such as Hillman River. This presents a very difficult situation for the responder. Again, if at all possible, it may be wise to let other EMS providers to take over as soon as those resources become available.

Any time that an EMS responder is called upon to treat family, friends, or coworkers, they are at risk for developing an acute stress reaction. The signs and symptoms of an acute stress reaction include a subjective sense of numbing or detachment, a decreased emotional response, depersonalization, difficulty concentrating, and feelings of guilt. This is often accompanied by extreme fatigue and a reexperiencing of the event through intrusive thoughts, dreams, and/or flashbacks (Thomas & Woodall, 2006). When this type of situation arises, it is wise to call for an additional EMS unit and a supervisor to the scene. The effects of acute stress can be minimized through the use of critical incident stress management (CISM). CISM involves various strategies, including an initial debriefing, the use of peer counseling, and follow-up with a licensed mental health professional. Supervisors would be wise to take the unit out of service for a period and assess the effects of the event on the EMS provider(s) who has been affected.

Lessons Learned

What Do You Know?

Volunteer firefighters in a small rural community responded to an attempted suicide at a neighbor's house. The patient was a 14-year-old boy whom the volunteers knew well. When they arrived, they were met by a police officer. They entered the house and saw that another officer was with the patient's parents. They entered the boy's bedroom and discovered his naked body on the bottom bunk of the bunk bed. He had tied a necktie around his neck and around the bed rail of the top bunk. He was hanging facedown. An adult magazine was on the bed below his face.

The boy had no pulse; his skin was pale, cold, and rubbery; signs of lividity were beginning to show. The volunteers determined that the boy had been deceased for some time and that there was nothing they could do. They debated about what to tell the parents. One of the firefighters wanted to call it a suicide. The police officer said it looked like a case of AEA. They decided to let the coroner determine the cause of death and did their best to console the grieving parents.

What Do You Need to Know?

It is essential for emergency responders to understand the concepts of crime scene integrity and evidence preservation. We are frequently called upon to treat patients who may be victims or perpetrators of a crime. Once we have concluded our treatment, law enforcement still needs to collect and document evidence. EMS is only one component of public safety. It is important that we respect the needs of other agencies and remember that we are part of a larger team.

EMS professionals are sometimes thrust into the role of having to tell someone that their family member is deceased. Every EMS responder should receive training in death notification, grief, and emotional first aid.

Resources

Law enforcement should be called to the scene any time a death has occurred. They will secure the scene and notify the coroner. In this case, grieving parents were to be considered. It is important to provide resources and to connect family members and friends to their social support system. This support system could include other family members, friends, church members, clergy, and/or co-workers. It is important to never leave someone alone after they have experienced the death of someone close to them. In this case, it would have been advisable to brief the Mulvaneys on what would happen next—what the role of the coroner is and what will happen to Kevin's body.

Responsibilities

Emergency responders are legally responsible not to disturb crime scenes and preserve evidence. We are also legally bound to protect the confidentiality of those we treat. Given the sensitive nature of this case, maintaining confidentiality is a critical component of customer service. We also have the responsibility to care for the family and friends of the deceased.

Action Plan

In this case, as in any other case, it is important to tell the family members the truth. Although nothing could be done to save Kevin, the actions of the emergency responders in this case will set the stage for how the Mulvaneys cope with the loss of their son. The volunteers or the police officers should stay with the Mulvaneys until someone else arrives. Before they leave, it would be advisable for the volunteers to take a set of vital signs and provide some emotional first aid. It is also important not to disturb the scene and preserve any evidence that may be present.

Justification of Your Action Plan

Preserving the scene is legally mandated. Providing care to the parents is simply the right thing to do. This is especially true in this case because they are their neighbors.

Follow-up

The responders in this case should also be aware of the effects that this type of call may have on them. It is important that they discuss the call afterward and they may want to consider a follow-up debriefing with both the police officers and the volunteer firefighters. Because this is a small community, it is unadvisable to discuss the call outside the group of responders. As such, it may be necessary to bring in someone from the outside to facilitate this process.

Because this is a small community, the responders will probably want to follow up with the Mulvaneys and express their condolences. Some responders may feel the need to attend the funeral, especially if they, or their family members, have a relationship with the Mulvaneys. It is appropriate for EMS responders to attend a funeral if they feel the need to.

Summary

Responding to fatalities is often one of the most difficult challenges in the EMS field. This is especially true when the decedent is a young person. Emergency responders must develop a set of skills to cope with these situations. These skills include preserving the scene, caring for the survivors, caring for each other, and caring for ourselves. Most people do not like to talk about death. Working in the EMS field means that we have to talk about it. We encounter it frequently and we do ourselves a disservice if we do not talk about it.

Caring for the grieving can sometimes be awkward. Emergency responders may not know what to say or how to say. Trust yourself in these situations. Most EMS professionals are caring and compassionate people. These are your best tools when caring for the grieving. Developing skills in the administration of emotional first aid can be a valuable tool and will serve you well throughout your EMS career.

Responding to fatalities reminds us that we are part of a comprehensive EMS system and part of an even larger public safety system. It is important that we remember our role in the system and respect the roles of others. This is best accomplished through strong interpersonal communication skills, interagency cooperation, and following the incident command system.

This case also illustrates the problems we encounter when we respond to someone we know. This could mean responding to friends, coworkers, or even family members. In most instances, we do not know this until we arrive on scene. The exception is when we have to treat one of our own who is injured or becomes ill at an emergency scene. Something to keep in mind is that after we have finished treating the patient, we become the customer. We are the ones who are in need of emotional first aid and CISM. Allowing ourselves to assume this role and make use of CISM will help us to cope with the stress and recover faster. It will also reduce the chances of developing chronic health problems related to job stress. It benefits every EMS agency to offer these services as part of the internal customer service.

Key Terms

Acute Stress Reaction   Symptoms that develop within 1 month after exposure to an extreme traumatic stress or event. These symptoms interfere with a person's daily functioning and are not the result of other psychological disorders.

AEA-Autoerotic Asphyxiation   Accidental death that occurs when an individual deliberately restricts the flow of oxygen to the brain while masturbating.

CISM-Critical Incident Stress Management   An adaptive short-term helping process that focuses solely on an immediate and identifiable problem to enable the individuals affected to return to their daily routine(s) more quickly and with a lessened likelihood of experiencing post-traumatic stress disorder.

Depersonalization   The sense of loss of self or of personal identity, sometimes referred to as the feeling of being on autopilot.

Detachment   The lack of feeling or emotional involvement in a problem, situation, or interactions with another person.

Emotional First Aid   A type of psychological intervention focused on helping a person to feel calm, safe, and well cared for during an acute, critical situation.

Incident Command System   A structured incident management system that is commonly employed at incidents in which span-of-control is an issue. The presence of an incident commander allows those treating the patients to focus on the task level, whereas the incident commander directs attention to strategy, safety, and resource management issues such as hospital and patient transportation availability.

Subintentional Death   Behavior that indirectly and/or unconsciously causes death.

References

Baker, S. P., O'Neill, B., Ginsburg, M. J., & Li, G. (1992). *The Injury Fact Book.* New York, NY: Oxford University Press.

Clark, M. (1996). The Autoerotic Asphyxiation Syndrome in Adolescent and Young Adult Males. Retrieved December 11, 2006, from http://members.aol.com/bj022038/AEA.htm.

Comer, R. J. (2007). *Abnormal Psychology,* 6th edition. New York, NY: Worth Publishers.

Jenkins, A. P. (2000). When Self-Pleasuring Becomes Self-Destruction: Autoerotic Asphyxiation Paraphilia. Retrieved December 11, 2006, from http://www.cwu.edu/~jenkinsa/aeaarticle.html.

Thomas, J., & Woodall, S. J. (2006). *Responding to Psychological Emergencies: A Field Guide.* Clifton Park, NY: Thomson-Delmar Learning.

14

Holiday Get-Together

Psychosocial, Ethical, and Leadership Dimensions

- Customer Service
- Mission Focus
- Community Relations
- Interpersonal Skills

Holiday Get-Together

Mr. Smith had been struggling with diabetes for the past 12 years. Most of the time, he was very good about watching his diet, monitoring his blood sugar levels, and taking his medication. Occasionally, something would happen to throw off his cycle and he would find himself having a reaction. Fortunately, his wife was always there to help him and these episodes were experienced as minor events.

It was Thanksgiving morning, and as was their usual practice, the Smiths sat down and ate breakfast together. This was the first time that Thanksgiving had been at their house in many years. They were both excited to see all of their children and grandchildren. Mrs. Smith spent the morning preparing the turkey. She was relieved that everyone would be bringing something and that she didn't have to prepare all the trimmings. Mr. Smith spent the morning bringing in extra chairs from the garage and setting up a card table for the kids.

The family started arriving around noon and everyone was happy to see each other. They had all become very busy the past few years and they just didn't get together as much as they used to. Everyone was in a good mood and having a good time. Mrs. Smith announced that dinner would be ready around two. The children all played in the yard, the women worked in the kitchen, and all the men settled down to watch football.

At 2:15 Mrs. Smith announced that dinner was ready. Everyone got up and headed to the table, everyone except Mr. Smith. He had fallen asleep in his chair watching football. His youngest son, Clifford, tried to rouse him. "Hey dad, wake up. Dinner is ready." Clifford gently shook him by the shoulder. Quickly, he realized that his father was not asleep; rather he was unconscious and not responding. "Dad! Dad! Wake up!" he shouted. Sensing that something was wrong, the rest of the family gathered in the living room.

"It's his blood sugar," shouted Mrs. Smith. "He didn't eat lunch when he was supposed to. Get me some orange juice!" She knelt down beside her husband. "John, wake up honey. John, wake up and drink some juice. John! John! Honey wake up! Oh god! Somebody call 9-1-1!" The call was placed and the family continued to try and wake Mr. Smith, but he was not responding. The family members were beside themselves.

Engine 14 pulled up in front of the Smith house just three and one half minutes later. It seemed like an eternity to the Smith family. The crew of four walked into the house and introduced themselves. Mrs. Smith explained her husband's condition and had Clifford retrieve his medication bottles. The crew went to work. One of the EMTs took a set of vitals and the other one tested his blood sugar level. His pulse rate was 100, respiration 24 and shallow, and blood pressure 128 over 90. His blood sugar level was 35. One of the paramedics started an IV and pushed D50. By this time, Ambulance 12 arrived on the scene. The second medic briefed the ambulance crew on Mr. Smith. Then one of the EMTs started the chatter.

"Hey how you guys been?" asked the firefighter/EMT. "Haven't seen you in a few days."

"Yeah, I know," responded the EMT from the ambulance. "We're doin' great."

"You guys had many calls today," asked the captain/paramedic.

"Not really, it's been kind of a slow day," responded the ambulance paramedic. "You guys been busy?"

"No, it's been slow for us too," answered the captain. "You guys been watching the game?"

"Oh yeah . . . hope we can make it back for the second half," shot back the ambulance EMT.

"What are you guys doing for dinner tonight?" inquired the engineer/EMT.

"We don't have any plans yet," answered the ambulance paramedic.

"Why don't you two come by the station later," invited the captain. "Sonny's been smoking a turkey since early this morning."

"That's sounds great!" the ambulance paramedic said enthusiastically.

By this time, Mr. Smith was starting to come around. The rest of the Smith family was not quite sure what to make of the situation. The chatter continued as if the Smith family was not there.

"Have you been out riding lately?" the firefighter/paramedic inquired of the ambulance EMT.

"No, I'm still waiting on those parts to get my bike fixed," replied the ambulance EMT.

"Those still aren't here!" exclaimed the firefighter/paramedic.

"No! Can you believe that?"

"I wonder what's taking them so long."

"Beats me."

"Well I was going to take the boys out to the dunes tomorrow. I've got that spare bike, why don't you come along?"

"Oh I don't know if I could do that."

"Sure! We'll have a great time."

Finally, Mr. Smith came around. The paramedics suggested that he should go to the hospital in the ambulance. His family agreed with the suggestion, but Mr. Smith said that he was starting to feel better. He indicated that all he needed to do was eat dinner and then his sugar levels would be back under control. The medics tried to convince him to go in, but he had been through this before. He asked to sign a refusal and told them that he would go in later if he started feeling bad again. The crews from Engine 14 and Ambulance 12 wished the Smith family a happy Thanksgiving and out they went.

Problem Solving

What Do You Know?

- Describe what you know about this incident.

What Do You Need to Know?

- What additional information would be helpful before further decision making?

Resources

- What potential resources would be helpful at this stage?

Responsibilities

- What legal, ethical, organizational, or interpersonal responsibilities should you consider?

Action Plan

- Decide what you would do next if you were in this situation.

Justification of Your Action Plan

- Explain the rationale you used for your decision.

Follow-up

- Would your action plan require any follow-up? Why or why not?

The Rest of the Story

The mood at Smith house was somewhat somber as the family sat down together for their Thanksgiving dinner. The family watched tentatively as Mr. Smith carved the turkey. As they began eating, they started to relax. They could all see that Mr. Smith was indeed going to be OK. The discussion at the table focused on what had just happened. The family described the behavior of the firefighters and the paramedics to Mr. Smith. They all agreed that they felt discounted and ignored. Mrs. Smith began to cry as she described the way she was treated. She felt belittled and disrespected. His mother's tears was all it took for Clifford to become angry. The next day he called the fire department to find out who responded the day before. He took down the names of the firefighters. His next call was to the ambulance company where he obtained the same information. He wanted to make sure he had every name right in the letters he would send to the fire chief and the president of the ambulance company.

Discussion

- What did the crews from Engine 14 and Ambulance 12 do right?
- What did the crews from Engine 14 and Ambulance 12 do wrong?
- Why do you think Mrs. Smith felt the way she did?
- What could the crews have done differently?
- If you were the supervisor processing Clifford's complaint, how would you handle this situation?

Skill Building

The members of Engine 14 and Ambulance 12 did arrive quickly to the scene and provided expeditious, definitive, and professional medical care. However, they breached some very basic yet important customer service protocols. Accomplishing the task at hand is not enough. Those we serve have come to expect, and rightfully so, compassion, focused attention, understanding of the significance of the event, all wrapped in a caring and professional attitude. Although it is true that all the emergency medical service (EMS) responders on the scene understood that the medical outcome of this particular call would be positive, they didn't acknowledge, through their actions, that the family did not share their confidence and were quite concerned. The crew members, especially the supervisors, should have recognized this call as one that required their collective efforts to extend excellent customer service. The entire family was present and their every move was being closely observed. Mrs. Smith felt discounted and disrespected by the casual conversations going on in her front room. Furthermore, the actions of the crew members probably made her wonder if her husband was getting all the attention he needed. Some excellent examples of sound and not so sound customer service practices can be found in Alan Brunacini's *Essentials of Fire Department Customer Service* (1996).

At the very least, those crew members not directly involved, or needed, in the treatment and care of Mr. Smith should have moved outside if a casual conversation was absolutely necessary. Actually, they should have refrained from unnecessary small talk and focused their efforts as reassuring the family members, especially Mrs. Smith.

Once Clifford filed his complaint with both agencies, the supervisory staff would be forced to act. When this behavior came to light, an investigation would probably ensue and the crew's previous actions would be examined. Was this an isolated incident or had this type of unprofessional behavior taken place in the past? No matter what disciplinary action would be necessary or recommended, this call should be treated as a learning moment. Not all scenes are alike. Not all scenes require the same degree of compassion and focused attention. However, all members on the scene should learn to recognize and understand the dynamics of each scene and act accordingly. Responders should always keep the "mission" in mind.

Lessons Learned

What Do You Know?

Engine 14, an Advanced Life Support (ALS) company staffed with two paramedics and two EMTs, has been called to a diabetic emergency involving an unconscious older male with a confirmed history of diabetes. They arrived, assessed the patient, and initiated treatment according to medical protocol. As the call progressed, the ambulance arrived and an informal conversation began between the emergency responders who were not directly treating and caring for the patient on the scene. The patient recovered consciousness and signed a refusal for further treatment and transportation to the emergency department. However, the patient's family was upset by the actions of the on-scene crews and filed a complaint.

What Do You Need to Know?

Useful information would include an understanding of the team dynamics of the engine and the ambulance crews. Is it a common practice for members of this organization to fraternize while on the emergency scene? Is the on-scene company officer an experienced supervisor? Any information that would assist in a better understanding of why these team members would engage in seemingly innocent yet damaging behavior would be useful. It would appear that the members not directly involved in the treatment of the patient did not focus on the important facets of community relations and customer service.

Resources

On-scene resources, in this case, were adequate. It could be argued that this scene had too many personnel, leaving several with the opportunity to engage in some unprofessional behaviors.

Responsibilities

Although legal and ethical standards are not at issue in this scenario, organizational and interpersonal responsibilities certainly are. When we are representing our department, agency, governing body, or company ownership, we are obligated to be professional; building a positive image for those we represent, providing sound customer service, and fostering feelings of good will result in excellent community relations. Interpersonally, we want those we serve to feel that we are focused on their needs, consider their situation as an important one, and never leave them feeling discounted or ignored.

Action Plan

In this case study, the damage had already been done by the time the emergency responders left the scene. The action planning would now include a mitigation plan designed to prevent this type of behavior in the future. If this was an ongoing problem, discipline may be necessary. If this was simply sloppy customer service and a case in which these individuals and their supervisor let their professional guard down, it might be time to revisit some concepts and constructs of sound customer service through training and education. This training could be as simple as bringing these folks together and having a little talk about the importance of staying focused on the mission and exhibiting positive regard, not only for the patient but for all significant others on the scene. The plan would also need to address the complaint filed by the patient's son. However, a formal complaint is not the sole reason this family should have been contacted. Even if a complaint had not been filed, they should be offered a formal apology from either the company officer or a representative of the fire department.

Justification of Your Action Plan

Though the crew's behavior was not intentionally malicious, it was harmful. Reasonable measures directed at ensuring that behaviors such as this would not be acceptable or perpetuated.

Follow-up

Follow-up would include the monitoring of this crew's on-scene behavior and checking in with the captain from time to time to re-inforce the lessons learned from this unfortunate encounter. Further follow-up in this case would probably include a letter of apology from the fire chief and the crew visiting the family and offering a formal apology.

Summary

The services we provide are often very intimate and personal. We are most effective when we are trusted and embraced. We build this trust and affection through consistently providing sound, professional, courteous customer service, staying consistently focused on our mission, and demonstrating unconditional positive regard by employing our interpersonal skills. By adhering to and believing in this philosophy, we will build relationship with our community.

We should always bring our "A" game to the scene regardless of the day of the week, the time, and the "holiday mode." Additionally, we should be aware that people from different cultures celebrate different holidays and also may celebrate and acknowledge traditional American holidays differently. Those we serve expect our best every time we respond. We must expect the same of ourselves.

Key Terms

Anxiety   A vague, unpleasant emotional state with the qualities of apprehension, dread, distress, and uneasiness.

Blood Sugar Level   The blood sugar level is the amount of glucose (sugar) in the blood. It is also known as serum glucose level. Normally, blood glucose levels stay within narrow limits throughout the day, but they are higher after meals and usually lower in the morning. In diabetes, the blood sugar level moves outside these limits until treated.

D50   Dextrose 50%. Class: Carbohydrate, hypertonic solution. The term dextrose is used to describe the six-carbon sugar D-glucose, the principal form of carbohydrate used by the body. D50 is used in emergency care to treat hypoglycemia and to manage coma of unknown origin.

Customer Service   The process and practice of delivering services. From the fire/EMS and EMS perspective, this is usually defined as the manner in which our services are delivered that produces a positive outcome.

Holiday Mode   Fire and EMS agencies develop individual cultures. Often Sundays and holidays are considered days in which the crews are allowed to relax more, plan their days, and generally recover from the rigorous Monday through Saturday schedule.

Professionalism   Actions in the workplace that exhibit high standards of performance, dedication, and commitment to the successful completion of a given mission.

Patient Refusal Form   A legal document utilized in the emergency medical field setting. By understanding and signing this document, the individual releases the responding individuals and their agency from any liability that may arise from the termination of their treatment and transportation to the emergency department. A "refusal of treatment and transportation" form must be signed by any patient not requesting transport by ambulance. If the patient is not capable of signing the refusal because of injury to their writing hand/arm, then the refusal must be witnessed. If the patient is not capable of signing the refusal because of an altered level of consciousness, you should reconsider whether they are mentally competent to refuse care.

Unconditional Positive Regard   Treating patients with respect and dignity and viewing them as worthy and capable, even when they do not act or feel that way.

References

Brunacini, A. V. (1996). *Essentials of Fire Department Customer Service*. Stillwater, OK: Fire Protection Publications.

15

Dog and Pony Show

Psychosocial, Ethical, and Leadership Dimensions

- Customer Service
- EMS Protocols
- Grief
- Death
- Interagency Cooperation
- Interpersonal Skills

▨▨▨▨ Dog and Pony Show

The dispatch "Channel six, infant code," jolted the crew awake just before the 7 am wake-up tone. The crew sprang out of bed, dressed, and ran to the truck. The engine company captain acknowledged their response and asked the dispatch to tell him what ambulance they would have and requested that an air ambulance be placed on standby.

Upon arrival, they were met at the front door by a young hysterical mother holding a month-old infant and a crying father. "We can't get him to wake up! We can't get him to wake up! I don't think he's breathing! Help us! Help us!" she screamed as she handed the swaddled baby to the first crew member through the door.

The paramedics sprang into action initiating PALS pediatric code protocols and the captain escorted the parents to the kitchen so that he could gather some information and get them out of the way. "I'm going to need to get some information from you folks. The paramedics are doing everything they can." As they walked into the kitchen, the paramedics initiated the assessment, established an airway, and started CPR. Kelly and Dave had worked together for several years and had the unfortunate experience of working several pediatric codes. If the baby had a chance, these seasoned paramedics were the right ones to have. It was at this point that the ambulance arrived to lend some much needed assistance.

Problem Solving

What Do You Know?

- Describe what you know about this incident.

What Do You Need to Know?

- What additional information would be helpful before further decision making?

Resources

- What potential resources would be helpful at this stage?

Responsibilities

- What legal, ethical, organizational, or interpersonal responsibilities should you consider?

Action Plan

- Decide what you would do next if you were in this situation.

Justification of Your Action Plan

- Explain the rationale you used for your decision.

Follow-up

- Would your action plan require any follow-up? Why or why not?

The Rest of the Story

Kelly and Dave were on the floor with the baby and the firefighter/EMT and the ambulance EMTs were bagging and providing compressions. "Dave, this little guy is gone. Look at his color. He's been down for quite a while, maybe for an hour or more," Kelly whispered.

"I know, I know but we've got to try. We've got to give this little guy a chance," Dave replied in a hushed tone.

The captain returned from the kitchen and leaned over so he could talk softly. "Hey guys. The last time the parents saw the infant awake was at his 4 am feeding. So we're dealing with anywhere from minutes to hours that he's been down. Also, she's had a difficult time having children and has had three previous miscarriages."

"That's what we figured Skip. We don't want to let him go but it looks pretty bad. Do you think we should call him?" Kelly asked.

"No!" Dave stated, raising his voice a little higher. "We might get lucky . . . and what about his parents? Are you ready to deal with everything that will happen if we call him now? I'm going to patch and see what the base hospital thinks we should do." Dave stepped outside the front door and patched with their base hospital. After what seemed like an eternity to the personnel working the code, Dave returned. "The ED said that given the baby's condition and the probable downtime, we could call him. I know this is fruitless but I don't want to deal with hysterical parents." Then he added, "Oh yeah, Howard is out front leaning his head against the rig. When we get a minute, someone needs to check on him."

"Listen, just listen for a minute," the captain said. "You guys keep at it and do everything you can. I don't think the parents are ready to deal with this, especially here in their home. Let's get him in the ride and I'll call the chaplain to meet us at the hospital. I'm not going to be the one to tell them, I don't get paid to be a grief counselor." With that he returned to the parents in the kitchen.

"He's right," Kelly stated. "Let's get him in the ride and you guys keep giving him CPR on our way." They reached the ambulance, loaded the gurney with the baby on it, hopped in, and discontinued all efforts at resuscitation while en route to the hospital.

Discussion

- Did these emergency medical service (EMS) professionals handle this situation properly?
- Is it OK to prolong the hopes of the loved ones through fruitless intervention when it is obvious that their loved one is deceased?
- What do you think was going on with Howard?
- What potential emotional needs should be addressed after this call is over?

Skill Building

Sudden infant death syndrome (SIDS) is the sudden and unexpected death of an apparently healthy infant who is under 1 year of age. Additionally, the cause of death cannot be explained after a thorough investigation that includes an autopsy, examination of the death scene, and review of the clinical history. The cause of SIDS is still unknown and there is no proven method for prevention. Some studies have identified risk factors for SIDS, such as putting infants to bed on their stomachs. The frequency of SIDS appears to be a strong function of the sex of the infant and the age, ethnicity, education, and socioeconomic status of the parents (Willinger, James, & Catz, 1991). According to a study published in October 2006 in the *Journal of the American Medical Association*, babies who die of SIDS have abnormalities in the part of the brain that helps control functions such as breathing, blood pressure, and arousal (Paterson et al., 2006).

EMS responders are often the patient's and family's last best hope. We are called on to intervene in situations where there is little hope of a positive outcome. The manner in which we handle these situations from the skills and interpersonal perspectives does make a difference to us, to the patient, and to those who love the patient. The EMS responder must be proficient in the area of skills application. This competency builds confidence and eases emotional stress as we know that all that could be done was done.

Evolving EMS field treatment protocols have shifted from the attitude that "we will work every code no matter what" toward a model that often requires the EMS responder to "call a code" in the field, under the supervision and advice of an emergency department physician. As this scenario demonstrates, pronouncing death in the field can be an extremely difficult thing to do. After all, we are the heroes. We are the good guys. We are there to make things better. Is it OK to continue the "dog and pony" show of cardiopulmonary resuscitation (CPR) and other invasive treatment so that we can avoid giving the family the bad news? This is a question that you and those you work with must answer. It is not a black-and-white issue and will change from situation to situation. Although excellent guidelines exist from the physical perspective, the actual calling of a code is more emotional than physical.

The captain in this case made the statement that he wasn't "paid to be a grief counselor." Although he may not see that as part of his profession, it is important for emergency responders to be aware of and respond to those who are experiencing a grief reaction. Grief is the intense emotional state associated with the loss of someone or something of significance. Every person will grieve in a unique and individual way. Grieving will be affected by each individual's own life history, and every person will grieve at a different pace (Thomas & Woodall, 2006).

The physical symptoms of grief can include heart palpitations, hypertension, and/or pressure in the chest. Muscular pain, headaches, dizziness, and confusion are also quite common. Individuals may also experience changes in appetite, sleep disturbances, and a general sense of fatigue. The psychological symptoms of grief include anger, anxiety, sadness, and/or despair. These may be accompanied by difficulty in concentrating and memory problems. Individuals who are grieving are also likely to experience feelings of loss, abandonment, loss of control, powerlessness, and/or helplessness (Thomas & Woodall, 2006).

EMS care for individuals experiencing grief should include a check of vital signs and the provision of emotional first aid. Emotional first aid is a type of psychological intervention focused on helping a person to feel calm, safe, and well cared for during an acute, critical situation. There are simple techniques that can be used to provide emotional first aid. The first technique is attending. These are behaviors that let the patient know that you are paying attention. They include maintaining good eye contact, using the patient's name, refraining from charting or taking notes, and giving the patient your full attention. The second technique is the use of open-ended questions. These are questions that cannot be answered by a simple yes or no. They are useful for gathering information. Noncommittal acknowledgments are actions that let the patient know that you are listening. They include nodding your head and vocalizations such as "ah," "uh-huh," and "hmmm." Responses such as "yes," "I'm listening," and "OK" are also helpful.

The use of "door openers" encourages patients to share more. Door openers are simple statements such as "tell me more," "help me understand that," or "explain that to me." Content paraphrases are remarks that let the patient know that you understand what has been said. This can be accomplished by simply summarizing what they have told you. One of the most difficult techniques of emotional first aid is the use of silence. Silence allows the patient time to collect his or her thoughts. Emergency responders should not feel like that they have to fill up the silence. If the silence is prolonged, try using an open-ended question. Self-disclosure can be effective techniques for letting the patient know what is happening for you at that very moment. Some examples are statements such as "I'm confused," "I don't understand," "I'm concerned about you," or "I want to help you." It is inappropriate and unprofessional for emergency responders to share personal stories from their personal lives.

Active listening is a more advanced technique in the provision of emotional first aid. Active listening involves listening for and identifying the emotional tone of what a patient is saying. Once the feeling is identified, it is reflected back to the patient in statements such as "you sound angry," "you're frightened," or "I hear sadness in your voice." Don't worry about always finding the correct feeling. If you identify the wrong feeling, the patient will simply correct you and the conversation can continue. Emergency responders should never tell patients that they do not feel the way they say they do. The final, and perhaps one of the most important techniques, is the provision of resources. A resource is any source of support or information that can be provided to the patient. It can be very helpful to develop or obtain a list of resources that is specific to your community (Thomas & Woodall, 2006).

Interpersonally, we must support each other in these emotionally charged instances. The patient's family is not the only group impacted by tragedy. It is important that we are aware of the different ways that different types of calls impact individuals on our team. It is important for the new EMS responders to discuss these types of scenarios in advance of being thrust into them. Talk with those who have had the experience.

Ask them to tell you about situations where they called a code and situations where they could have called a code but chose not to. Also, ask them about how they emotionally cope with the sadness and tragedy they witness. Most importantly, when you've experienced these types of incidents firsthand, make sure that you self-evaluate and watch for signs of a critical incident stress reaction. Symptoms of a stress reaction can include changes in personality, mood swings, difficulty in sleeping, and difficulty in concentrating. Symptoms may also involve changes in eating habits, significant weight gain or loss, problems with personal and professional relationships, and/or substance abuse.

Supervisors should be trained to recognize the symptoms of stress reactions. Employees who are experiencing stress exhaustion should be given the option of voluntary referral to seek professional help. An employee assistance program is a good resource if one is available. Supervisors may make a mandatory referral if stress reactions are negatively impacting job performance. EMS agencies should have a critical incident stress management (CISM) program in place. A good program will utilize a combination of trained mental health professionals and peer support. Every member of the CISM team should receive initial training and continuing education. The CISM team should be called when an agency experiences a critical incident. Employees involved in the incident should be taken out of service. The CISM team should provide an initial defusing. Participation in a defusing should always be voluntary. A more formal debriefing may be held within a day or two of the incident. Debriefings should only be conducted by those trained to do so. The term *debriefing* has become much maligned. It may be wise for an agency to select different terminology (Thomas, 2006).

Lessons Learned

What Do You Know?

An ALS crew has been dispatched to an infant code just before 7 am. Upon arrival, they encountered two distraught parents. The mother was holding the limp infant and she immediately handed the male infant to the first paramedic through the door.

The crew initiated pediatric advanced life support (PALS) code protocols as the captain took the parents into the kitchen to gather more information. The captain talked with the parents gathering some medical history and went back to the crew working on the infant and shared the collected information, including that the family had not seen the baby responding for 3 hours. The paramedics informed the captain that the baby's chances of survival were extremely unlikely. Even though it would have been entirely logical, the captain and the crew decided to continue their efforts to save this child. This decision was made, primarily, in the hope of a miracle and for the parents' benefit. Secondarily, the crew did not feel prepared to deal with all of the emotional turmoil that pronouncing this baby dead would bring to the scene. They continued to work on the infant code until the ambulance doors were closed and they were on their way to the hospital.

What Do You Need to Know?

From a medical standpoint, all the required patient information is known. However, it is also necessary to understand the EMS protocols and the process of providing emotional first aid.

Resources

When death occurs at the scene of a medical or traumatic event, it is always the best practice to call for law enforcement. Unfortunately, many apparent SIDS deaths have turned out to be crime scenes. We should always acknowledge that we are not professional investigators and/or crime scene investigators. When requesting law enforcement to come to our scene, we are not accusing anyone of anything and not condemning the survivors but we are simply following standard operating procedures and EMS protocols.

Even though the patient has not been pronounced, or "called," on the scene, it would also be the best practice to get other resources en route to the scene if time permits. This crew requested that the fire department's chaplain be dispatched to the receiving hospital. It may have been a good idea to have him respond to the scene. Furthermore, the captain may have asked the parents if there was anyone they would like to contact. For example, grandparents, brothers, and sisters can be very helpful in stressful situations such as this. This couple may have had a pastor, priest, rabbi, or other spiritual advisor whom they may want to be with them during the early stages of their grief. We are advocates not only for the patient but also for those near and dear to the loved ones of the victim or patient.

Responsibilities

Legally and ethically, this crew would have been well within bounds if they chose to call the code on the scene. However, when examining this scenario from the organizational and interpersonal perspectives, some important responsibilities are worthy of note. This crew represents a helping organization. The services provided are more than technical; they are very personal. Emergency medical responders often see, and serve, people during the most emotionally and physically stressful times of their lives and the lives of those they love. It is important that we act in ways that exhibit empathy, sympathy, and compassion.

Interpersonally, we have the responsibility to communicate those feelings of understanding and act in professional ways. We must always be present for those we are helping, actively listening to what they are saying and also observing how they are doing. It is also important to serve as advocates. It is our responsibility to anticipate their real and potential needs. It is through this practice that we can bring all the necessary and available resources to the scene or to the hospital in an effort to assist the living in respecting and grieving the dead.

Action Plan

An action plan similar to the one implemented by this crew is very sound. Like most emergency calls, this call was not perfect. In the dynamic environment of EMS, perfect may not be a realistic goal.

We do the best we can with what we have, always seeking new, innovative, and creative ways to best meet the challenges we encounter. We learn from experience and we learn from others, including those we serve.

The baby has been transported and will soon be pronounced dead. The crew could wait at the emergency department for the parents to arrive and express their condolences, restock, regroup, and go back to service. This may be a good idea and can often prove empathetic. It's one thing to show you care during the "what-if" phase through professional actions and interventions. It is human to show you care after all efforts have been exhausted.

Justification of Your Action Plan

Of course all action plans should be planned and implemented with the law, agency's standard operating procedures, and EMS protocols as the foundation. A good plan with a good outcome is often not enough if these important considerations are breached. These regulations are in place for a reason and for the most part have been tested over time. In this case, these benchmarks were adhered to. Always start a plan from the perspective of what you are allowed to do, then move to what should we do.

Follow-up

Depending on the personal and professional experience of this crew, the supervisor may want to initiate an informal or formal debriefing process. In this scenario, Howard was experiencing some difficulty with the emotions this call elicited in him. At the very least, the captain should check in with him before shift change.

The informal process may be as simple as keeping the company out of service for a while, perhaps getting something to eat and drink and sit down and touch base with each other. In a situation like this in which the crew was probably getting off after returning to quarters, it is probably prudent to get them together before leaving quarters and returning to their other lives.

The formal critical incident stress debriefing varies in style and availability depending on the agency. If this resource is available in your agency, all the organization's members should be aware of it, understand what it is for, and how to utilize it for self and others.

Summary

Every EMS professional will experience the seemingly meaningless death of children and infants. These types of responses will always be difficult from the skills and emotional perspectives. Every current or aspiring EMS responder should expect to work with the dead or nearly dead and be prepared to experience the grief suffered by those near and dear to the patient or victim.

The challenge to those choosing this line of work is to stay healthy and human. It is true that we often must mask our immediate feelings and emotions while helping those in need, remaining calm and professional, while we may be coming apart inside. This often does not come without a cost. It is important to understand this aspect of the job and to make conscious efforts to remain physically and mentally healthy. However, it is our ability to empathize, sympathize, and understand what loved ones are experiencing during and after the death of a loved one. In fact, these are the very qualities that make us human in this humane business. It is when these feelings are not present that we should worry.

During these kinds of emotionally stressful calls, it is very important to return to the basics, following our EMS protocols, standard operating procedures, and operating within the law. Additionally, we call on our interpersonal skills to address the emotional and physical needs of our patient and the patient's loved ones. Efforts grounded in these principles will always lead to positive customer service outcomes.

Key Terms

Anxiety   A vague, unpleasant emotional state with the qualities of apprehension, dread, distress, and uneasiness.

Active Listening   Listening for and identifying the emotional tone of what a patient is saying. Active listening includes reflecting the feeling back to the patient. If you are incorrect, the patient will correct you. Examples include "you sound angry," "you're frightened," and "I hear sadness in your voice." It is important to never tell a patient that they do not feel the way they say they do.

Attending   These are behaviors that let the patient know that you are paying attention to them. Examples of positive attending behaviors include maintaining good eye contact, using the patient's name, refraining from charting or taking notes, and giving the patient your full attention.

Content Paraphrase   Remarks given to the patient that let him or her know that you understand what they have been saying. Some suggested techniques include summarizing what the patient has told you and using quotes if appropriate.

Critical Incident Stress Management   It is an adaptive short-term helping process that focuses solely on an immediate and identifiable problem to enable the individuals affected to return to their daily routine(s) more quickly and with a lessened likelihood of experiencing post-traumatic stress disorder.

Despair   An emotional state characterized by the loss of all hope or confidence.

Door Openers   Comments that encourage the patient to share more information. Examples include "tell me more," "help me understand that," and "explain that to me."

Emotional First Aid   A type of psychological intervention focused on helping a person to feel calm, safe, and well cared for during an acute, critical situation.

Employee Assistance Program   A benefit program provided by the employer who usually offers assessment, short-term counseling, and referral services.

Noncommittal Acknowledgments   Actions that let the patient know you are listening to them. Examples include nodding your head while the person is talking, vocalizations such as "ah," "uh-huh," or "hmmm," and responding with comments such as "yes," "I'm listening," or "OK."

Open-Ended Questions   These are useful for gathering information regarding the emergency. A good method to use when asking an open-ended question is to ask questions that require more than a simple yes or no answer—"tell me what has happened to you today." This method encourages patients to talk freely.

Providing Resources   The conscious and specific actions taken by an individual or an advocate to call for and secure the resources that are necessary to successfully mitigate a situation.

Self-Disclosure   Disclosing to the patient what is happening for you at that very moment. Examples include "I'm confused," "I don't understand," "I'm concerned about you," and "I want to help you." It is inappropriate and unprofessional to share personal stories from your life.

Silence   Allowing time for silence allows the patients the time to collect their thoughts. It is not necessary to feel as though you must fill up the silence. However, if the silence is prolonged, try an open-ended question.

Stress Reaction   Emotional and physical reactions that are manifested because of experiencing or being exposed to a disturbing and/or harmful event.

SIDS–Sudden Infant Death Syndrome   This is a syndrome marked by the symptoms of sudden and unexplained death of an apparently healthy infant under 1 year of age. The term *cot death* is often used in the United Kingdom, Australia, and New Zealand, whereas the term *crib death* is used in North America.

References

Paterson, D., Trachtenberg, F., Thompson, E., Belliveau, R., Beggs, A., Darnall, R., Chadwick, A., Krous, H., & Kinney, H. (2006). Multiple Serotonergic Brainstem Abnormalities in Sudden Infant Death Syndrome. *JAMA* 296(17).

Thomas, J. (2006). *EMS Providers.* Lecture at Arizona State University, Tempe, AZ.

Thomas, J., & Woodall, S. J. (2006). *Responding to Psychological Emergencies: A Field Guide.* Clifton Park, NY: Thomson-Delmar Learning.

Willinger, M., James, L. S., & Catz, C. (1991). Defining the Sudden Infant Death Syndrome (SIDS): Deliberations of an Expert Panel Convened by the National Institute of Child Health and Development. *Pediatric Pathology* 11, 677–84.

The Coke Scandal

Psychosocial, Ethical, and Leadership Dimensions

- Ethics
- Team Dynamics

The Coke Scandal

Bill and Ted swung their ambulance into the parking lot of a fast-food restaurant hoping to catch a quick lunch between calls. The morning had been steady but not overly busy. Bill ordered a cheeseburger, fries, and a large drink. Ted also chose the cheeseburger and fries; however, he asked for a glass of water. After picking up their orders from the counter, they walked over to the soda fountain to fill their cups. Bill filled his cup with ice and put it under the Coca-Cola dispenser. Ted also filled his glass with ice and Coca-Cola.

The two medics sat down at a table to enjoy their lunch. They made small talk discussing the morning's calls and each other's plans for the coming weekend. Before they left, they both went back to the soda fountain and refilled their cups with Coke. After they had gotten back into their rig, Bill turned to Ted and said, "Dude, that stunt you pulled in there was really not cool."

"What stunt? What are you talking about?" asked Ted

"The Coke."

"Huh?"

"You ordered the same thing I did, except you asked for H_2O. Then you filled up your free cup with Coke."

"Yeah . . . —so."

"That is so totally not cool."

"I saved a dollar-sixty-nine!"

"It's not about the money dude. We are both wearing uniforms and driving an ambulance. What if somebody saw you do that and decided to narc? Not cool!"

Problem Solving

What Do You Know?

- Describe what you know about this incident.

What Do You Need to Know?

- What additional information is required before further decision making?

Resources

- What potential resources would be helpful at this stage?

Responsibilities

- What legal, ethical, organizational, or interpersonal responsibilities should you consider?

Action Plan

- Decide what you would do next if you were in this situation.

Justification of Your Action Plan

- Explain the rationale you used for your decision.

Follow-up

- Would your action plan require any follow-up? Why or why not?

The Rest of the Story

Bill and Ted continued arguing about the soft drink.

"Why are you hassling me about this?" complained Ted. "It's just a freakin' Coke!"

"I don't want to get busted for this dude," countered Bill. "I like this job, and besides it helps me get lots of babes."

"You're right about that," grinned Ted. The two exchanged a high five.

"I think you should still go in and pay for it."

"No way dude! What if they, like, call our boss or something? We'd be so busted."

"Good point," agreed Bill while shaking his head up and down.

"Let's get out of here before somebody else figures it out."

"Yeah, let's go save some more lives." With that, Bill shifted the ambulance into drive and pulled out of the parking lot.

Discussion

- Did Ted's actions violate any laws and/or professional ethics or community standards? Why or why not?
- Did Bill's actions violate any laws and/or professional ethics or community standards? Why or why not?
- Suggest some ways in which Bill and Ted could have resolved this situation in a professional manner.
- Discuss the standard to which emergency responders are held in your community. Are these expectations realistic?
- What do you do when offered free drinks when in uniform and on duty?
- What would you have done if Ted were your partner?

Skill Building

Ted's actions in this case are common. Perhaps some of us have even done it ourselves. Ted's actions constitute pilfering (stealing in small quantities). And yes, it is against the law. The reason that people feel like they can get away with it is because the likelihood of prosecution is small. A soda fountain in a fast-food restaurant functions on the honor system. The community standard is that customers pay for their drinks. Many establishments allow patrons to refill their cups for free if they have paid once. Fast-food restaurants are aware that the pilfering of soft drinks takes place. However, they trust that most citizens are honest and will pay for their drinks. The consequence of people pilfering from the soda fountain is that the price of the drinks will eventually go up.

What is unique about this situation is that Bill and Ted were both in uniform and were in a marked ambulance. Any time we are in uniform, we must be fully cognizant of the fact that we represent not only the agency we work for but also the entire emergency medical service

(EMS) profession. Emergency responders are granted a high degree of public trust. We are allowed entry into homes and businesses and are given carte blanche to do what needs to be done. This may include opening cabinets and drawers to look for medications. We open purses, wallets, and/or briefcases to search for identification. We ask questions of a highly personal nature and are told information that individuals would not disclose to just anyone. Bill and Ted's actions not only reflect badly upon themselves but also create a stain of dishonor on the entire EMS profession and erode the public's trust.

It is usual for vendors to offer firefighters and EMS personnel free drinks and/or food while they are in uniform and on duty. Many agencies feel this is OK and it represents a way that the community can show their appreciation. A policy stating whether this is acceptable or unacceptable will be agency specific and personnel should consult with a supervisor and the policy before encountering this in the field.

Those we serve have a right to expect a high standard of integrity and honesty from EMS personnel. Our collective actions define who we are and the standards we represent. These actions, whether in uniform, out of uniform, on duty, or off duty, also serve to build the public's confidence is us. It is through this confidence that patient care is enhanced.

Bill's comment about how the job gets him "lots of babes" reflects a sexist attitude and displays a level of emotional immaturity. Even though the partners were alone, the comment tells us a great deal about Bill's worldview.

EMS training and education programs should incorporate material focusing on attitude, professional standards, and decorum. When outlining these expectations, the prospective emergency medical technician (EMT) or paramedic candidate will better understand the profession and be better prepared to determine whether this job is right for them. Hiring processes and practices should be evaluated to determine whether candidates are properly screened for dedication and commitment to the profession as well as for maturity and professionalism.

Finally, those in charge of staffing crews should always seek to match crew partners with several factors in mind. Sound practice would include matching experience with inexperience, younger with older, and seasoned and tested with potential immaturity. In essence, crews should be set up with professional growth in mind, providing the younger-newer crew member with a good example from the perspectives of skill enhancement and positive customer service.

The EMS professional will more than likely encounter behavior that is counter to their values and morals. In this scenario, Bill could have returned to the restaurant and paid for the drink remarking that his partner had simply forgotten to pay. Bill could also use this situation as an opportunity to set some basic partner ground rules regarding their expectations of each other.

Lessons Learned

What Do You Know?

Two paramedics stopped to eat at a fast-food restaurant. One of the partners took his water glass to the soda dispenser and filled up his cup with Coke. Once they got back to the rig, Bill informed Ted that it was not acceptable to take a drink that he had not paid for. Bill further informed Ted that they were in uniform and representing their agency and what Ted had done was, in essence, stealing. They briefly discussed whether Ted should go back and pay for the drink but decided not to and drove off.

What Do You Need to Know?

It was obvious that at least one of the crew members knew that this was wrong and unprofessional. It would be helpful to know if these paramedics had received any type of ethics, community relations, or professional development training. When preparing what, in this case, would be an "after-action" plan, some information about previous types of and frequency of similar incidents during their employment with this company could provide insight as to whether this was an isolated incident or one incident in a series of problems.

Resources

Resources, in a scenario such as this, should be utilized in a proactive rather than reactive fashion. As mentioned earlier, are the actions an issue that can be addressed through training? Is this a case of a bad partner matchup? Is this a case of poor or inadequate supervision? Or, is this an issue of poor morale? Whether Ted's actions were exacerbated by one or all the above, he has a problem. Should this problem be allowed to continue, it will more than likely progress to actions of a more serious nature, resulting in discredit to himself, his partner, the agency he works for, and the entire EMS community. In an effort to prevent this type of behavior from occurring again and possibly becoming more serious, the key resources would be peer pressure, supervision, training, and disciplinary action.

Responsibilities

The bottom line is that what Ted did was stealing; it is illegal and unethical. His actions placed his and his partner's job in jeopardy. Though his theft was low on the financial scale, it was high on the scale that damages public trust, undermines community relations, and creates embarrassment for the organization he represents. Interpersonally, we all share responsibility for those we work with. Whether we acknowledge it, our actions in the workplace do influence those on our team. Our actions can be influential in a positive or negative way.

Action Plan

Incidents such as this occur when controls are not in place to prevent them. Therefore, action plans directed at preventing this type of behavior before it can occur include training and orientation that clearly delineates duties, responsibilities, and expectations. The next level of training and supervisory instruction would include sessions on ethics, community relations, and building the trust of the public we serve.

Although this incident more than likely went unreported, it does prove that this kind of behavior can take place. An action plan that incorporates proactive rather than reactive measures would definitely be the most beneficial approach for all parties involved.

Justification of Your Action Plan

Proactive measures directed at preventing an event from occurring are always more effective and beneficial than consistently being forced to implement reactive measures.

Follow-up

Had the incident been reported and consequently acted upon through the chain of command, some follow-up would be required. The supervisor would want to monitor the actions and movements of the crew and would probably be smart to assign Bill and Ted to different, more mature partners.

Summary

The effectiveness of the services we provide relies heavily on possessing the trust and good will of those we serve. We go into people's homes, vehicles, offices, and other places of business unmonitored. We work on people when they are unconscious and vulnerable. It is paramount that we constantly and consistently monitor and modify the way we act and speak while in public. Finally, if we are to be trusted with their safety and lives, we should always want to be above reproach.

Key Terms

Pilfering   To steal small amounts or trivial objects.

Professional Ethics   Ethical positions in the workplace. A person's professional ethics are influenced by personal philosophies, beliefs, morals, and those they work with and for.

Public Trust   The foundation of those that govern and those who serve in the public's interest. This trust is earned through honesty, integrity, hard work, professionalism, and the delivery of competent service.

Crass Course

Psychosocial, Ethical, and Leadership Dimensions

- Diversity
- Interpersonal Skills
- Sexual Harassment
- Team Dynamics

░░░░░ Crass Course

Amy and Lou had been working on the ambulance together for almost 2 years. Amy was just beginning her career as a paramedic and Lou was a veteran of 15 years. Amy really appreciated the mentoring and guidance she received from Lou. He was an excellent teacher and she felt they made a good team. Their agency provided all the Advanced Life Support (ALS) response for their county so there was no shortage of opportunity for her to practice her skills.

It was late afternoon when they were dispatched to a motor vehicle accident on County Road 14, east of the Harwell Dairy. This was a long way away and it took them a while to get there. The only other information they could get from the dispatcher was that it was a head-on collision, there were multiple patients, and the local fire department was on scene. The long response gave Amy time to think. "It must be bad if they are calling for us," she thought to herself. "It's after school. I hope it's not kids from the high school."

When they arrived, they could see that a pickup truck had crossed the centerline and collided with a motorcycle. There was one fire truck and a sheriff's deputy on the scene. Amy and Lou got out of the ambulance, gathered their gear, and walked up to the scene. The captain informed them, "There were two people on the motorcycle. They are both in bad shape. The guy in the truck is drunk. He's a little banged up, but seems OK. The sheriff has him right now."

Lou radioed dispatch and requested another ambulance. He and Amy both knew that it would take a while for the second ambulance to get there. They split up and both began working on one of the patients from the motorcycle.

Amy's patient was a young woman in her mid-twenties who had been riding on the back of the motorcycle. It appeared as though she had been launched off the back of the motorcycle and had landed in the middle of the road. Fortunately, she was wearing a helmet. A firefighter was holding traction on her neck and had stabilized the airway.

Amy found that she was conscious, moaning, and complaining of pain in her leg. Amy completed her assessment and determined that she had likely fractured her left femur. She decided to start an IV. She got the bag ready and asked the captain to hold it while she started the line. The captain stood next to her and held the IV bag as she knelt down next to the patient and inserted the needle. After getting it started, she turned to adjust the flow and inadvertently found herself staring into the captain's crotch. Nothing could have prepared for what happened next. The captain moved his hips and thrust his pelvis into Amy's face.

Problem Solving

What Do You Know?

- Describe what you know about this incident.

What Do You Need to Know?

- What additional information would be helpful before further decision making?

Resources

- What potential resources would be helpful at this stage?

Responsibilities

- What legal, ethical, organizational, or interpersonal responsibilities should you consider?

Action Plan

- Decide what you would do next if you were in this situation.

Justification of Your Action Plan

- Explain the rationale you used for your decision.

Follow-up

- Would your action plan require any follow-up? Why or why not?

▓▓▓▓▓ The Rest of the Story

Shocked and taken aback, Amy was not sure what to do next. She looked at the captain and he was just smirking at her. Amy did the only thing that she knew to do. She continued working on the patient and getting her ready for transport. Lou had radioed for a helicopter to transport the motorcycle driver. The second ambulance had arrived and was assessing the driver of the pickup truck. Amy's patient was loaded into the back of her ambulance and Lou drove them to the hospital.

After they had finished at the hospital, Lou could sense that something was bothering Amy. They reviewed that call and he assured her that she had done everything by the book and had quite probably saved the woman's life. Still, he sensed that something was wrong. He pressed and eventually Amy confided what the captain had done to her. Outraged and angry, Lou assured her that she hadn't done anything wrong and that the captain's behavior was unacceptable. He told her that they would have to call a supervisor. Amy was reluctant. "We have to work with these guys," she told him. "I can get over this. I'll be OK."

Lou was persistent. He explained that she was right. They would have to work with those guys again and that is exactly the reason that they needed to do something about it.

"Look, I got into this job knowing that things like this could happen," countered Amy. "I don't want to be the cause of any problems."

"You are not the problem. He is!" Lou radioed dispatch. He took the ambulance out of service and requested that a supervisor meet them at quarters. The supervisor listened to what had happened. He asked both Amy and Lou to write down what had happened. The ambulance service contacted the fire department and filed a complaint. Eventually, the captain was disciplined for his behavior. Amy was not looking forward to the next time they would have to respond with that captain.

Discussion

- Should Amy have done anything different on scene?
- What was wrong with the captain's behavior?
- Do you think this is an example of sexual harassment?
- How would you handle the situation if you were the captain's supervisor?
- What kind of message does the captain's behavior send to his crew?

Skill Building

The captain's behavior is clearly unprofessional and uncalled for. According to the Equal Employment Opportunity Commission (EEOC), sexual harassment takes place when there is a violation of a trusting relationship that should be sex neutral. The captain's actions were uninvited, unwanted, and unwelcome. These elements are vital to determine whether behavior constitutes sexual harassment (Edwards, 2005). Fire and emergency medical service (EMS) professionals must have the confidence that they will not be subjected to such behavior within their agency or from the employees of other agencies with whom they respond.

Amy was certainly placed in a difficult position. She was treating an immediate patient with potentially life-threatening injuries. Had she chosen to confront the captain on scene, it is possible that his behavior could have become the focus and taken the focus off of patient care. Furthermore, because there were few responders actually on scene, Amy needed the help of every responder who was there. It is hard to know what the captain would have done had she confronted him. At the same time, it is important for any individual who is being harassed to set boundaries and let the harasser know that the behavior is unwelcome. This could have been done on scene with a look, a nonverbal cue, or a short statement such as "knock it off." In any case, Amy should have reported the incident to her partner and to her supervisor.

Behavior such as this has no place in emergency services. The captain's supervisor should take some type of disciplinary action. The type of action will depend on the captain's history and if there have been previous incidents. At the very least, the captain should receive a written reprimand and quite possibly a period of probation. Sexual harassment is a very serious issue and the captain put his entire fire department at risk for adverse legal action. It may also be prudent for the fire chief to send a formal letter of apology to the head of the EMS agency and to Amy.

This case reflects the fact that there are those in fire and EMS who struggle with gender and other diversity issues. Changes occurring in the workforce result in the fact that the number of women and ethnic minorities entering the fire and EMSs is steadily increasing. The advantages of a diverse workforce far outnumber those of a nondiverse workforce. Those advantages include more alternatives and perspectives when problem solving, greater opportunity to discover information or find significant mistakes, increased innovation, and a greater diversity of skills and abilities. It can also lead to an improved quality of work and an increased ability to serve a diverse community (Thomas, 2005).

Lessons Learned

What Do You Know?

Two paramedics from the county EMS department were dispatched to a motor vehicle accident. When they arrived, the county sheriff and the local fire department were already on scene. The medics were informed that a pickup truck had crossed the centerline and collided head-on with a motorcycle. The pickup truck driver was drunk and was a delayed patient. There were two riders on the motorcycle and both were immediate patients.

The female paramedic began treating the woman who was riding on the back of the motorcycle. She started an intravenous (IV) line and asked the fire captain to hold the IV bag. When she turned to adjust the flow, she found herself at eye level with the captain's crotch. The captain responded by thrusting his pelvis into Amy's face. Amy ignored the behavior and continued to treat her patient.

After the call was over, Amy reluctantly shared her experience with her partner. Her partner responded by taking their unit out of service and requesting a meeting with a supervisor. After discussing the incident with the supervisor, the two medics documented everything that had happened. The EMS department filed a complaint with the fire department and the captain was disciplined.

What Do You Need to Know?

Every employee should be educated on the issue of sexual harassment. This training should include a review of the agency's policies on harassment and the proper procedures for reporting harassment.

Resources

Employees should have access to a policy manual. If harassment occurs, employees should follow the chain of command and notify their supervisor. If the supervisor is the person perpetrating the harassment, the employee should notify that person's supervisor. If there is no further option up the chain of command, the employee should notify the human resources department.

Responsibilities

Sexual harassment is a violation of federal and state law. It is also likely to be a violation of an EMS agency's policies. Employees have an obligation to report if they are subjected to harassment or if they are a witness to harassment. If employees witness harassment and fail to report it, they themselves run the risk of being charged with harassment.

Action Plan

An employee who is being sexually harassed should notify a supervisor immediately. After making the notification, they should take the time to document the incident. The same is true for any employee who bears witness to sexual harassment.

Justification of Your Action Plan

Sexual harassment is illegal and is a policy violation.

Follow-up

Any case of harassment is likely to trigger an investigation. Employees should fully cooperate with the investigation. Management should move swiftly to protect employees who are being harassed and put an end to the behavior.

Summary

Sexual harassment is an example of one type of harassment. Harassment can occur in many forms. When harassment takes place, it begins to damage the morale of an agency. Emergency responders frequently work long shifts in close quarters with their coworkers. To do their job at the highest level, it is important that they feel safe and comfortable. Harassment erodes at the feeling of security and destroys working relationships. If left unchecked, it will eventually lead to decreased patient care and poor customer service.

Changes in our society mean that there is greater diversity in the EMS workforce. It also means greater diversity in the communities that we serve. A good EMS professional is respectful of those differences. If we allow members of our profession to treat others poorly, we help to create a blemish on the entire field of EMS and diminish the public trust.

Key Terms

Equal Employment Opportunity Commission   The federal agency responsible for ending employment discrimination in the United States.

Immediate Patient   A patient who requires rapid assessment and medical intervention for survival.

Sexual Harassment   Unwelcome attention or behavior of a sexual nature.

References

Edwards, S. T. (2005). *Fire Service Personnel Management*, 2nd edition. Upper Saddle River, NJ: Prentice Hall.

Thomas, K. (2005). *Diversity Dynamics in the Workplace*. Belmont, CA: Thomson-Wadsworth.

18

Cat on a Hot Tin Roof

Psychosocial, Ethical, and Leadership Dimensions

- Interpersonal Skills
- Psychological Emergencies

Cat on a Hot Tin Roof

It was a beautiful spring day. The ladder crew had only run a couple of calls. The crew was feeling pretty relaxed, the truck had been washed, they had finished cutting some practice ventilation holes down at the fire department training facility in the morning, and they even had some time to work out. It was late afternoon and they were looking forward to catching the end of the ball game on television. Just as they were settling in, a rescue call came out for a child trapped on a roof.

The crew darted out to the truck and began responding Code 3 to a residence in a middle-class inner-city neighborhood. No further information was available from dispatch. Not sure what was happening, the captain urged the engineer to get there quickly. When they arrived, a frantic mother met them at the curb.

"He's up there!" she cried out.

The crew looked up in disbelief to see a 12-year-old boy riding his BMX bike up and down the valleys on the pitched roof of a two-story house. They quickly went for the ground ladders as the captain walked over to the house with the mother.

"How did he get up there?" the captain asked.

"I don't know," replied the mother. "I told him to get down, but he won't. He has ADHD. I called his psychologist and he told me to call you."

"We'll get him down," reassured the captain. "What's his name?"

"His name is Brad," declared the mother.

As the firefighters approached with the ladder, the captain called up to Brad and asked him what he was doing up there.

"I'm riding my bike," was the matter-of-fact answer.

"Your mom says it is time to get down," implored the captain. "We are coming up to get you and your bike down."

"Leave me alone. I am not coming down," was Brad's retort.

"See what I mean," complained the frustrated mother.

The captain repeated his words. "We are going to get you down."

Brad was defiant. "If you come up here, I am going to ride my bike off the edge."

Problem Solving

What Do You Know?

- Describe what you know about this incident.

What Do You Need to Know?

- What additional information is required before further decision making?

Resources

- What potential resources would be helpful at this stage?

Responsibilities

- What legal, ethical, organizational, or interpersonal responsibilities should you consider?

Action Plan

- Decide what you would do next if you were in this situation.

Justification of Your Action Plan

- Explain the rationale you used for your decision.

Follow-up

- Would your action plan require any follow-up? Why or why not?

The Rest of the Story

Considering Brad's threat to ride off the edge if they tried to bring him down, the captain quickly abandoned his plan to go up on the roof with a ladder. Instead, he sent the youngest firefighter on his crew up to a second-floor bedroom with a window that opened to the roof. It turns out that this was Brad's room and that he had pushed his bike out the window to get it on the roof. The firefighter talked to Brad through the opened window but did not go out onto the roof. He asked Brad about his bike and where else he liked to ride it. He also asked Brad about what kind of music he liked, what movies he had seen lately, and who were his favorite sports teams. In total, the firefighter spent 15 minutes talking with Brad before he convinced him to come back in through the window.

Discussion

- Was this an appropriate call for the fire department?
- What were the safety issues in this situation?
- Do you think that 15 minutes was too long to spent trying to talk him down?
- What might have happened if the captain persisted in his plan of going up on the roof with a ladder?

Skill Building

Sometimes firefighters are asked to intervene in situations that are psychological or behavioral in nature. In some circles, a call like this may not even be considered a "true" emergency. However, Brad was in a dangerous situation and the fire department did have a duty to act. It is our job to respond when the public calls and not to make judgments about what is and isn't an emergency and to use all the time required to reach a successful outcome.

Attention-deficit disorder (ADD) is a chronic neurological condition that is usually present since birth. It is often, but not always, accompanied by hyperactivity, this is known as attention-deficit hyperactivity disorder (ADHD). Symptoms of depression are common with both ADD and ADHD. Those with this disorder are easily distracted, disorganized, and forgetful, have difficulty following instructions, and are inattentive to details. Additionally, and pertinent to this case study, is the impulsivity that is often present. Simply put, impulsivity is acting without thinking first. This disorder is usually medicated with central nervous system (CNS) stimulants and antidepressants (Thomas & Woodall, 2006).

The actions of the responding crew were appropriate but may have been improved through a consultation with Brad's psychologist. The mother had just recently contacted him so an additional phone consult between the psychologist and the captain may have proved beneficial. Fortunately, the captain chose to not aggressively attempt to remove the boy from danger. The selection of the nonintrusive method of talking Brad down by utilizing the youngest crew member was wise. The young firefighter was able to build rapport with Brad as he talked his language and engaged him at his level. Admonishment and lecturing would have been a dangerous mitigation strategy possibly leading to a bad outcome for all.

Lessons Learned

What Do You Know?

A fire department ladder crew was dispatched to a call for a child trapped on a roof. When they arrived on scene, they found a 12-year-old boy riding his bike up and down the pitched roof of the house. The mother explained that she had tried to get him down but he refused. She further reported that he was being treated for ADHD. She had spoken to his psychologist who suggested she call the fire department.

The captain initially tried to send his crew up on the roof using ground ladders. When they attempted to do this, the boy threatened to ride his bike off the edge of the roof. The captain changed his strategy and sent the youngest firefighter on the crew up to a second-floor window to talk with the boy. The firefighter was eventually able to persuade the boy to come down from the roof.

What Do You Need to Know?

It is important to recognize that sometimes situations that at first seem trivial and insignificant have the potential to quickly become very serious. This emphasizes why it is important to do a good scene size-up. Factors to consider are the type of roof construction, the roofing material (shingles, tiles, etc.), the time of day, and the weather conditions.

Fall injuries are the leading cause of nonfatal injury-related emergency department visits and are the most common cause of traumatic brain injury. Falls over 10 feet are considered to be potentially fatal (National Center for Injury Prevention and Control, 2006).

Resources

Because of the high potential for injury in this situation, it may be wise to request the presence of a supervisor or a law enforcement officer. They can serve a number of roles including safety officer, crowd control, and as a witness in the case of fall. From the risk management perspective, having a witness is a wise precaution. This protects both the emergency responders and the agency from possible litigation.

In this case, the boy's psychologist is also a possible resource. The psychologist may be able to provide some background information that could be helpful. He also could have given insight into whether the boy was suicidal. Some jurisdictions also have units that specialize in psychological and behavioral emergencies.

Responsibilities

The fire department has the responsibility to see that this boy comes down from the roof. Although he was not suicidal, his behavior did represent a danger to himself.

Action Plan

Talking the boy down from the roof is the best strategy in this case. It is important for the firefighters to remain calm. Their calm demeanor will help to calm the mother down and keep the boy for escalating his behavior.

Justification of Your Action Plan

Talking the boy down is the strategy with the least amount of risk. Had the captain insisted on sending firefighters up the ladder, he risked the boy following through on his threat to ride off the edge. In addition, any firefighter going up on the roof becomes at risk for injury.

Follow-up

The boy was already in treatment with a psychologist, so no referral is indicated. The ladder crew might have to review safety procedures and document the incident.

Summary

This call is an example of the importance of taking the time to think through an intervention strategy. In this case, the captain was willing to spend the time talking the boy down. A more aggressive approach may have lead to injury or death. It is easy to rush into action, particularly when the task seems simple, routine, or mundane. Taking the time to do a good scene size-up and assess the scene is crucial for a positive outcome.

The firefighter talking with Brad in this case exhibited strong interpersonal skills. By taking the time to build a rapport and have a conversation with the boy, he neutralized a potentially dangerous situation. Several key factors must be a part of every patient contact. Always introduce yourself and state why you are there. Some patients may not be in a state to recognize or correctly interpret the meaning of a uniform. Treat patients with unconditional positive regard. That means being respectful, not making judgments, and understanding that it is truly an emergency to them. Building trust and rapport can be accomplished by showing empathy for the patient's situation, being supportive and reassuring, and displaying a calm, compassionate, and caring attitude.

Key Terms

Antidepressants   A class of psychotropic medications, or other substance such as an herb or nutritional supplement, used for alleviating the symptoms of depression.

ADD/ADHD   A neurological condition that is characterized by distractibility, forgetfulness, hyperactivity, and impulse control.

CNS Stimulants   Psychotropic medications that speed up physical and mental processes.

Unconditional Positive Regard   Treating patients with respect and dignity and viewing them as worthy and capable, even when they do not act or feel that way.

Scene Size-up   The process of assessing the emergency scene for potential hazards to ensure the safety of all patients and emergency responders at the scene and assessing the nature and type of emergency.

References

National Center for Injury Prevention and Control (2006). *Injury Topics and Fact Sheets.* Atlanta, GA: Centers for Disease Control.

Thomas, J., & Woodall, S. J. (2006). *Responding to Psychological Emergencies: A Field Guide.* Clifton Park, NY: Thomson-Delmar Learning.

19

All Dressed Up and No Place to Go

Psychosocial, Ethical, and Leadership Dimensions

- Customer Service
- EMS Protocols
- Mission Focus
- Patient Advocacy

All Dressed Up and No Place to Go

Harriet just wasn't feeling right. At the age of 85, the days that she was feeling bad seemed to outnumber the days that she felt good. She had followed her usual routine: toast and decaf for breakfast, and waiting 30 minutes after her breakfast to take her medications. She couldn't put her finger on it, but something was just not right. Being the compliant soul that she was, she always followed her doctor's orders. "The doctor told me that if I wasn't feeling right I should come in," she thought out loud to herself. "He said that if there wasn't anyone around to help during one of my spells that I should call 9-1-1? Yes that's what he said," she stated, again talking to herself out loud.

She looked for Margaret, her agile and active 74-year-old next door neighbor. She was always willing to give her a ride to the hospital. This time, Margaret was nowhere to be found. "Probably, at jazzercise or out square dancing again," she thought as she shuffled about her morning routine. "Well, I guess it's time to call an ambulance for a ride to the hospital. Wait, I can't go in looking like this. I don't think I need a shower but I most certainly must pack a bag and get dressed." She went about her business, fed the cat, got dressed, and packed her suitcase. When she was done with all these tasks, she sat down in the kitchen, picked up the phone, and dialed 9-1-1.

"Channel 6-ill woman. 14356 W. Sunset Drive, Ambulance 12."

"Well here we go again. Wonder who's not right today," said Terry, a 5-year veteran EMT.

"Really," replied Sharon, the ALS provider on Ambulance 12. "Should be Sunset Acres not Sunset Drive. Can you believe how many old people are moving in there lately?"

As they approached the address, Sharon shouted, "Oh my God can you believe this? She's standing at the curb, fully dressed, and carrying a suitcase! I've got to take a vacation. This is getting to be too much for me!"

Problem Solving

What Do You Know?

- Describe what you know about this incident.

What Do You Need to Know?

- What additional information would be helpful before further decision making?

Resources

- What potential resources would be helpful at this stage?

Responsibilities

- What legal, ethical, organizational, or interpersonal responsibilities should you consider?

Action Plan

- Decide what you would next if you were in this situation.

Justification of Your Action Plan

- Explain the rationale you used for your decision.

Follow-up

- Would your action require any follow-up? Why or why not?

The Rest of the Story

Sharon and Terry discussed what they should do. Terry chuckled and said, "She looks like she's waiting for a taxi to take her to the airport." Together they agreed that they would do a thorough assessment before deciding what actions to take.

"Good morning ma'am," said Sharon. "What seems to be the problem today?"

"I'm just not feeling right. I need to go to the hospital. My doctor said I should go to the hospital when I'm not feeling right."

"OK," responded Sharon. "Is there a specific problem you are having?"

"No," said Harriet. "I just don't feel right."

"All right, do you mind if we take a look at you?" asked Sharon.

"That's fine, but I just need to go the hospital," replied Harriet.

Sharon and Terry did their assessment and couldn't find anything significant. Harriet's vital signs were normal, she was alert and oriented, and she did not have any specific pains or problems that could be identified. Harriet reported that she took her daily medication according to the doctor's instructions. Terry contacted the base hospital and apprised them of the situation. After consulting with the physician, Harriet was transported to the hospital Code 2 (no emergency lights and no siren).

Discussion

- Did Harriet do anything wrong?
- Did the crew do anything wrong?
- In view of the growing geriatric population, can this scenario be viewed as an increasing problem?
- Did Harriet's physician do anything wrong?
- What kinds of problems did the transport of Harriet create for emergency departments?
- What can be done to address this challenge on the response, community, and health service provider's levels?

Skill Building

Some might say that Harriet's actions are an abuse of the emergency medical service (EMS) system. What Terry and Sharon didn't know is that before she called 9-1-1, Harriet did try to get a ride from her neighbor. In her mind, Harriet was merely following her doctor's orders. By being cooperative and compliant, she readied herself for the trip so that it would be easier for the ambulance to just pick her up. She thought that she was showing respect for the ambulance crew.

Although they expressed some frustration and exasperation between themselves, Sharon and Terry did a good job of treating Harriet with respect and dignity. They followed all the necessary protocols by completing a thorough assessment and consulting with their base hospital. It would be easy to criticize them for their attitude as they got the call and drove up to the scene, but it is important to note that they kept their personal feelings separate from their patient care and acted in a very professional and compassionate manner.

Because we don't really know what condition Harriet was being treated for, it is hard to second-guess her physician. Many healthcare providers instruct their patients to call 9-1-1 in the event of an emergency. Unfortunately, many people lack knowledge regarding what is truly a medical emergency. Therefore, they dial 9-1-1 for what they perceive to be an emergency. It is important to remember that in their mind they perceive the situation to be a true emergency. And finally, many view 9-1-1 as the normal way to access medical attention.

In Harriet's case, it is clear that her condition was nonemergent. Perhaps Harriet could benefit from some education regarding when to use 9-1-1 and what other transportation alternatives are available to her. It is also possible that Terry and Sharon could have arranged alternative transportation if it was available in their community.

The transport of nonemergent patients does place a burden on the emergency medical service (EMS) system. It takes emergency responders out of service for more serious emergencies and congests already busy hospital emergency departments. At the same time, it is important to remember that the EMS is just one part of a larger healthcare system. For various reasons, some members of our community have no other alternative but to use EMS as their primary healthcare provider. These reasons can include, but are not limited to, poverty, lack of insurance, lack of transportation, lack of a social support system (i.e., family and/or friends), limited intellectual resources, and substance abuse.

It is the role of EMS providers to service the population in every instance. The EMS Systems Act of 1973 legislated that there must be adequate means to transport patients to the nearest appropriate medical facility in every community (Walz, 2002). The Consolidated Omnibus Budget Reconciliation Act (COBRA) of 1985 requires all emergency departments to provide services regardless of a patient's ability to pay (Walz, 2002). If the EMS system were to make the provision of service conditional, it would certainly erode public confidence and public support. That is why it is incumbent on EMS providers to provide the best possible customer service on each and every call.

EMS systems and the healthcare systems in general can take a number of steps to reduce the number of nonemergent calls to 9-1-1. Most public safety agencies have created 24-hour nonemergency numbers. This provides the public access to the EMS system for nonemergency health issues or other issues unrelated to EMS. This was done to try and curb the misuse of the 9-1-1 system. Many jurisdictions are also beginning to implement 3-1-1 as the nonemergency number. Pathway management is a process created by healthcare agencies that are outside the EMS system. This system allows patients to have access to a trained healthcare professional who can assess their condition and make recommendations. Sometimes the recommendation is to access the EMS system, but more frequently patients are directed to urgent care or other healthcare options. Public education also plays a role in addressing this issue. For instance, "Make the Right Call" is a public education program sponsored by the National Highway Transportation Safety Administration. Its goal is to educate the public when it is appropriate to call 9-1-1 and when it is not (Walz, 2002).

Lessons Learned

What Do You Know?

A two-person advanced life support (ALS) ambulance has been dispatched to attend an ill woman in a neighborhood that is becoming known as a retirement community. As they arrived, they saw an elderly woman standing at the curb with a small overnight bag apparently waiting for transportation to the hospital. They agreed in advance to do a thorough medical assessment and did just that even though they found nothing remarkable or life threatening. After consulting with the base hospital, they transported her Code 2.

What Do You Need to Know?

There is really not much more to know. One can assume that Harriet was utilizing the EMS system in a manner that reflected how she thought it was to be used. In her mind, she was being compliant with her doctor's instructions. Apparently, she had not been instructed in alternative, nonemergent transportation options and may not have had money to call a cab.

Resources

If this encounter was to be approached from an educational perspective, alternative hospital transportation options could be discussed with Harriet. Talking to a customer about alternative hospital transportation options does not come without risk. As EMS responders, we want to be very careful about giving people the impression that we do not want them to call us. This may create a reluctance to call 9-1-1 when a true emergency exists. This task is probably better referred to the receiving hospital's social worker in hopes of identifying an alternative nonemergent transportation resource(s) with the premise that Harriet had not done anything wrong but rather there may be a better way to accomplish the same goal.

Responsibilities

We have the legal responsibility to respond when called always keeping in mind that what we define as an emergency and what a caller defines as an emergency may be very different. We have the training, expertise, and experience to help us define what is emergent and what is not. Those we serve usually do not possess the same knowledge base from which to make a decision. Ethically, we have the responsibility to respond to all emergencies with the same commitment to excellence, professionalism, and efficiency, and we would if we were called to assist a member of our family. Our organizations have equipped us, trained us, supported us, and paid us often with the tax money paid by those we serve. We use our skill set and interpersonal skills to successfully mitigate the problems we are called to solve, building customer rapport, customer goodwill, and community relations with one patient at a time.

Action Plan

The action plan implemented by this crew was sound. Even though the crew had some misgivings about why a nonemergent person would call 9-1-1, they maintained their professionalism, handling themselves well and representing their agency and the EMS community in a positive manner.

Justification of Your Action Plan

Any action plan based on the patient's best interest, even though in this case there really was not a patient per se, has a solid foundation and a good chance of ending in a positive outcome. Although we do not know the actions they took upon arrival at the emergency department, it would have been prudent of them to share their experience with the hospital's social worker in hopes of finding Harriet a more appropriate transportation resource.

Follow-up

Follow-up in this scenario would only be required if the action plan incorporated the services of the hospital's social worker. Had those services been utilized in the hopes of assisting Harriet, the crew would want to check in and determine the outcome of that consult.

Summary

This story exemplifies the need to view and assess our systems through the eyes of those we serve. The number of what could be considered nonemergent calls for service are increasing and all emergency medical response agencies should make every effort to educate the public on the proper utilization of our services. Additionally, alternative, nonemergent transportation resources should be identified and readily on hand.

Key Terms

Customer Service   The process and practice of delivering services. From the fire/EMS and EMS perspective, this is usually defined as the manner in which our services are delivered that produces a positive outcome.

Nonemergent Patients   Those individuals who have accessed the EMS or medical system for medical attention but whose illness or injury is not life threatening.

Pathway Management   This is a process created by healthcare agencies that are outside the EMS system. This system allows patients to have access to a trained healthcare professional who can assess their condition and make recommendations.

Public Education   Comprehensive wellness and injury prevention programs designed to eliminate or mitigate situations that risk the lives or health of the public.

References

Walz, B. (2002). *Introduction to EMS Systems*. Clifton Park, NY: Thomson-Delmar Learning.

20

Food Poisoning

Psychosocial, Ethical, and Leadership Dimensions

- Diversity
- Interpersonal Communications
- Team Dynamics

Food Poisoning

Engine 6 just finished loading the hose back on the truck. They had spent the morning conducting their annual hose test. Every member of the crew was tired and sweaty. They were looking forward to taking showers and sitting down to lunch. Because all the hose was back on the truck, the captain placed the crew back in service. It only took 10 minutes for the first call to come in, ... abdominal pain. The engine took almost 2 minutes to respond because the engineer and one of the two medics were both in the shower when the call came out.

The engineer dried off quickly and threw on his physical training uniform and a pair of EMS pants. He was standing next to the truck putting his boots on when the medic emerged still drying her hair with a towel. They responded quickly to a private residence in a socioeconomically depressed part of town. The information on the mobile data terminal indicated that the patient was a 14-year-old female. The crew determined en route that their female medic would examine the patient.

They were met at the door by the mother who was flanked by two little boys. She was holding an infant in her arms. In what could best be described as Spanglish, the mother explained that her oldest daughter had been home sick for the past 2 days. She had been unable to eat and was complaining of severe abdominal cramps. The crew was directed into a back bedroom where they found the girl lying on her back covered with blankets.

The engineer started to take a set of vital signs while the female medic began to interview the girl. The girl spoke good English but was very pensive and anxious. The engineer reported that the girl's blood pressure was elevated, her pulse was rapid, and her breathing was quick and shallow. The mother tried to explain that she thought her daughter had got food poising from the cafeteria at school. When the female medic asked for permission to examine the girl, she became very panicky and scared. Sensing that something was not right, the captain asked the mother if she would go with him and take the boys into the living room.

Upon physical examination, it was clearly evident that the young girl was about to become a mother herself. The girl confided to the medic that she knew she was pregnant but didn't think she was due for several weeks. She thought this was simply the routine cramping that she had been experiencing throughout the pregnancy. She also stated that her mother did not know she was pregnant.

Problem Solving

What Do You Know?

- Describe what you know about this incident.

What Do You Need to Know?

- What additional information would be helpful before further decision making?

Resources

- What potential resources would be helpful at this stage?

Responsibilities

- What legal, ethical, organizational, or interpersonal responsibilities should you consider?

Action Plan

- Decide what you would do next if you were in this situation.

Justification of Your Action Plan

- Explain the rationale you used for your decision.

Follow-up

- Would your action require any follow-up? Why or why not?

The Rest of the Story

The engineer walked out into the living room and whispered in the captain's ear that they were about to deliver a baby. He then walked out of the front door to get the obstetric kit and the pediatric bag off the truck. The captain, not knowing that the mother was unaware of the pregnancy, smiled and said, "Congratulations! You're about to become a grandmother."

Discussion

- What did the crew do right in this scenario?
- Where did things go wrong with this call?
- Did the engineer in this case do anything wrong?
- Did the captain in this case do anything wrong?
- Was there a violation of the patient's right of confidentiality?
- How could this situation have been handled differently?

Skill Building

The crew in this scenario did several things right. They allowed the female paramedic to take the lead in assessing this patient. This is an example of doing some preplanning on the way to a call and capitalizing on the strengths of any given crew member. The captain also did the right thing by asking the rest of the family to step into the living room while his crew worked on the patient. Often this allows the patient to disclose sensitive information. This also shows concern for patient modesty and privacy. Additionally, it allows the family members to calm down and gives them the opportunity to ask questions and express their concerns. Family members may also be willing to provide additional information that they would be reluctant to share in front of the patient.

This call is also an example of how a simple communication breakdown can have disastrous consequences. If the engineer had also whispered to the captain that the rest of the family was unaware of the pregnancy, the situation could have been handled with more tact and discretion. Had the captain been given all the information, he could have avoided an awkward and embarrassing situation. He might have been able to pull the mother aside and explain to her what was happening in private. Another solution would have been to ask the patient if she would like a few moments with her mother to explain what was happening. Protocols would have insisted that the female paramedic remain in the room, but it would have allowed the mother to receive the news in a more personal way. It may also be prudent in some situations for the crew, or partners, to huddle together and determine the best course of action.

Patient confidentiality with adolescents can be a tricky situation. Some states allow adolescents to seek medical care without parental consent. This is especially true when it comes to emergency medical care. Most states consider a minor to be emancipated when he or she becomes a parent. It is important for responders to be aware of the laws that govern patient confidentiality in their jurisdiction.

Lessons Learned

What Do You Know?

Engine 6 was dispatched to attend a call for abdominal pain. En route they were informed that the patient was a 14-year-old girl and they decided that their female medic would take the lead. The crew was met at the front door by the girl's mother and younger brothers. Upon the start of the examination, it was evident that the girl was very anxious and nervous. Sensing this, the captain led the mother and her brothers into the living room. Upon further examination, the medic discovered that the girl was pregnant and was about to deliver. The girl stated that she knew she was pregnant but that her mother did not know. As the engineer went out to get the proper equipment, he briefed the captain on the fact that they were going to deliver a baby; however, he neglected to tell his captain that the mother did not know about the pregnancy. Not knowing this, the captain blurted the information out to the mother.

What Do You Need to Know?

EMS providers need to be aware of their state laws regarding parental consent for treatment, particularly when it applies to teenagers. They should also be aware of patient confidentiality and Health Insurance Portability and Accountability Act (HIPAA) laws.

Resources

Given the fact that this is a teen birth, the crew might want to request an ambulance and an additional paramedic unit. It might also be wise to request that an air transport be put on standby in the event of serious complications. Although it was not the case in this story, the captain might want to consider requesting law enforcement. This would be a wise precaution in the event that the parent, sibling, or boyfriend became upset and agitated upon learning of the pregnancy.

Responsibilities

Because the 14-year-old girl becomes emancipated when her child is born, she now has legal right to give consent and make treatment decisions for both herself and the newborn infant. This could prove awkward and may be difficult to explain to the 14-year-old's mother.

Action Plan

The crew should continue to treat the patient and deliver the baby. The captain should remain with the mother and try to keep her calm. Depending on the mother's reaction to the news, the captain might want to call his supervisor and let him know about the situation.

Justification of Your Action Plan

The crew is clearly obligated to continue care despite the communication error. The captain may want to let a supervisor know just in case there is a problem later. At that point, the supervisor can make his or her decision about whether to respond to the scene.

Follow-up

After this call is over, the crew may want to discuss teamwork and communication. The captain should also brief his supervisor and document what had happened as there is the potential for a citizen complaint.

Summary

This case demonstrates how a small error in communication can lead to a serious mistake. When making a report, EMS professionals should make a point to include all the information that they have. It is better to provide more information than is needed than to omit a key fact. Incomplete reports can lead to problems with patient care, scene safety, etc.

The crew in this case showed great sensitivity to their patient's modesty needs. EMS providers should examine patients in private and out of the view of others whenever possible. If not possible, the EMS provider should provide a sheet, a gown, or some other garment to preserve modesty where it is appropriate.

The fact that this call happened in an economically disadvantaged part of the town with citizens who are not part of the dominant culture bears examination. One has to wonder if this crew took a more cavalier attitude because of the part of town they were in. They may have made the mistake of stereotyping or prejudging this family. It is important for emergency responders to treat every citizen with the same degree of respect and professionalism regardless of their personal characteristics or life circumstance.

Key Terms

Confidentiality   Federal law requires that all patient information and patient records be kept confidential.

Discretion   The quality of being discreet, especially with regard to speech or behavior.

HIPAA   This act established regulations for the use and disclosure of protected health information.

Parental Consent   Laws that require one or more parent's permission notification before their minor child can legally engage in certain activities such as seeking health care.

Patient Modesty   Respecting the needs of patients who need to be undressed for examination or need to disclose sensitive information.

Spanglish   A blend of the English-language words for Spanish and English. It is a dialect in which the speaker intermittently changes from Spanish to English and vice versa.

21

A Few Good Men

Psychosocial, Ethical, and Leadership Dimensions

- Ethics
- Community Relations
- Interpersonal Skills
- Diversity

A Few Good Men

Ambulance 44 was located in an upscale neighborhood with long curving drives lined with palm trees and wide sidewalks. The two-person paramedic crew enjoyed the neighborhood they served and often took advantage of the amenities like the country club swimming pool and the tennis courts. They also appreciated that they frequently slept all night and only rarely had to run into the inner city. The four or five calls a shift that they did run were usually BLS and again these rarely occur after midnight.

Around 10 pm, they were aroused by dispatch informing them to respond to an ill woman not too far from the station. Conversation during the response was limited to directions and the nature of the call. With no real sense of urgency, the ambulance pulled up to the house. They grabbed their gear and walked up the long driveway. A distinguished middle-aged man with dark hair and a touch of gray on the sides answered the door. "Her name is Suzanne and she's in the master bedroom down this hall and to the left. I can't figure out what's wrong with her but I know she needs your assistance."

"Thank you sir," the senior paramedic responded. "We'll take a look."

The situation took an unexpected turn when they entered the bedroom. Suzanne was lying on the opulent king-sized bed and was propped up by pillows. She was clad in a see-through "Teddy" that left much of her legs uncovered. She was an extremely attractive, slim, and tanned woman in her late forties or early fifties.

"Oh hello gentlemen, Harold told me you were coming. I hope we didn't wake you."

"No, you didn't bother us at all Mrs....? I'm paramedic Jackson. My partner and I are here to take care of you," he stated as he turned to his partner and suggested, "Mike, can you see if you can find her a blanket?"

"The last name is Johnson; please call me Suzanne and a blanket will not be necessary," she coyly replied.

The partners were starting to get a read on the situation and Jackson asked Mike to call for the husband. "I'll be right in. I'm just refreshing my drink," Harold informed Mike.

Jackson started his assessment by asking the patient the usual questions. "Where do you hurt? What seems to be the problem? Do you have a fever? Do you have a headache?" He ran through a litany of questions for which she would only provide vague answers.

It was then that Harold returned to the doorway of the bedroom. He walked in, sat his drink down on the bedside table, and slipped off his robe exposing his naked body. He very casually and nonchalantly laid his robe on the bed and stated, "So, who would like to go first? Suzanne and I would like to provide you both with a bit of entertainment tonight."

Jackson looked at Mr. Johnson and politely said, "Could you give us just a minute?" Jackson waved Mike into the hallway for a quick conversation.

Problem Solving

What Do You Know?

- Describe what you know about this incident.

What Do You Need to Know?

- What additional information would be helpful before further decision making?

Resources

- What potential resources would be helpful at this stage?

Responsibilities

- What legal, ethical, organizational, or interpersonal responsibilities should you consider?

Action Plan

- Decide what you would do next if you were in this situation.

Justification of Your Action Plan

- Explain the rationale you used for your decision.

Follow-up

- Would your action plan require any follow-up? Why or why not?

The Rest of the Story

Once in the hallway, Jackson stated, "Sorry Mike but this just isn't right. Nothing but bad things can come out of this. I suggest we get out of here ASAP. Let me handle it."

Jackson returned to the bedroom and politely stated, "We're sorry Mr. Johnson but were not going to be able to stay. We appreciate the invitation but we're on duty and need to be available for other emergencies." That said, they picked up the gear and made their way out to the ambulance. They returned to quarters without saying much and when they got back they just went back to bed.

Discussion

- What did the paramedics do right in this scenario?
- Should a supervisor be notified?
- Would you document this call?
- If you did document this call, how would you do it?
- How would you handle a situation like this if you were dispatched to the Johnson's home again?
- What actions should be taken at the administrative level?

Skill Building

Jackson and Mike made the right decision in choosing not to participate in the couple's plan. They did, however, make two very serious errors: one, not completing an encounter form, and two, not notifying a supervisor. A record of Ambulance 44 being dispatched to this address for an ill woman exists. This record includes the time of dispatch, on-scene arrival, and departure time. Without an encounter form, a record of patient contact does not exist. It is true that there really wasn't a patient and an assessment did not take place, but even these facts were not documented. By not immediately notifying a supervisor, the medics have placed themselves in potentially deep trouble if the couple decided to turn the situation around and file a formal complaint.

Had Jackson and Mike decided to complete an encounter form, it should have included that the patient was found sitting in the bed, speaking in full sentences, alert, and capable of answering questions. Additionally, the form would document that no chief complaint was identified by the patient and no further assessment or treatment occurred.

When the crew got back in the ambulance, they should have immediately gone out of service, requested dispatch to have a supervisor meet them either at their quarters or another location. It is important to go out of service and meet at a location other than the Johnson's home. Going out of service is necessary as this situation requires immediate action and should not wait for any reason. Staying at the Johnson's and asking a supervisor to respond there would probably bring undue attention from the neighbors and could very well make the Johnsons uncomfortable, suspecting that this situation might be going in a direction that could damage their reputation and standing in the community.

By taking immediate action, Jackson and Mike would have initiated a series of events that would ultimately protect them, their agency, and the local governing body. The administrators of the agency would want to know about this call, the actions taken, and the subsequent documentation. They, in turn, would send this up the chain of command until it reached the agency head. The agency head would then notify the appropriate governing official. In the interest of patient confidentiality, the patient's name would not necessarily need to be provided. The report passed up to the governing body would probably only include the scenario encountered and how it was handled. This is also important if this incident resulted in a formal complaint from the Johnsons. If the Johnsons decided to notify a council person, mayor, or city manager of a different but plausible scenario that would place Jackson and Mike in the wrong, the agency head would be notified immediately. By being made aware of this in advance by Jackson and Mike, the agency head and those above would be better prepared to deal with the situation.

In addition to handling the immediate situation, the agency administrators may want to 'flag' this address with the stipulation that a supervisor automatically be added to any future dispatches to this address. Responding personnel should be briefed that the agency would respond to future calls for service to this address, render care to those in need, and be respectful and courteous to any and all present.

Lessons Learned

What Do You Know?

We know that a two-person, advanced life support (ALS) ambulance crew was dispatched to a private residence for a reported ill woman. Upon arrival, they were met at the door by a person whom they probably considered the husband of the reported ill woman. He directed them to the bedroom where they encountered a middle-aged scantily clad, attractive woman. During the thorough medical assessment, the husband propositioned the two crew members offering the sexual favors of his wife. The crew politely refused and then excused themselves from the scene.

What Do You Need to Know?

This is a pretty straightforward scenario. The patient's nonemergent status had been confirmed. The motivation as to why they were called to the scene had been established, and although the outcome was initially positive, that outcome remained dynamic and it could be assumed that the trouble may not have been over.

Resources

The need to notify a supervisor was noted earlier, emphasizing the desire not to make a scene out of an uncomfortable situation. The notification of the next higher level of supervision, for advice and direction, represents the best strategy to deal with this situation in the short and long run.

Responsibilities

Legally, this crew was probably on sound footing. They had done nothing illegal. Ethically, they had a duty to respond and did so. Furthermore, they held to their ethical obligation regarding professional behavior, performing their duties in a professional manner and not engaging in a sexual encounter.

Mike and Jackson represented their organization professionally, although calling a supervisor and completing an encounter form would have protected their company and themselves to a greater degree. They also demonstrated considerable interpersonal skills as they politely and professionally extricated themselves from a very uncomfortable and delicate situation.

Action Plan

The action plan initiated by these paramedics, although spontaneous by circumstance, was effective and probably did produce a positive outcome. However, as noted in the discussion, there were some oversights that could have some negative consequences.

Justification of Your Action Plan

The actions taken in this scenario were based on sound ethics and professional practice. The paramedics were courteous and did not belittle or chastise the Johnsons for their inappropriate proposal. As noted in the discussion, they may have fallen just short of handling this situation in the best possible manner, but they did lay a sound foundation for a long-term successful solution through their initial actions.

Follow-up

In this instance, no news would, in fact, be good news. If the Johnsons didn't counter with a complaint to the city or ambulance company, everything would most likely be fine. This does not, however, mean that follow-up and follow-through would not be a good idea. If this happened once, it could happen again, if not with the Johnsons then with someone else. Proactive measures such as those mentioned in the discussion should be explored and potentially implemented.

Summary

When in doubt, return to the basics, follow EMS protocols, complete all required documentation, and report unusual situations to the next level of supervision. Ground your decisions is solid professional and personal ethics. Seek to always enhance community relations and use your interpersonal skills to your personal and professional advantage. We will often encounter folks who hold a different set of values and morals—be aware that this diversity exists and be prepared to effectively deal with circumstances that will tax your personal and agency resources.

Key Terms

Encounter Form The patient charting form utilized to document patient contact, medical findings, medicines, chief complaint, and other important information utilized by the receiving hospital in an effort to understand the situation and expeditiously treat a patient. This form is also used to document a coherent patient's right to refuse treatment and transportation to a medical facility. Although the content requirements of this document can vary from agency to agency, it is a legal document.

Appearances

Psychosocial, Ethical, and Leadership Dimensions

- Community Relations
- Internal and External Communications

Appearances

The Glen Valley Fire Department was recruiting for an upcoming entry-level firefighters test. They anticipated hiring 25 recruits for the upcoming academy class and things were in full swing. Interested candidates were encouraged to visit Glen Valley fire stations, ride along, and learn about the job, the department, the city, and those whom they may soon be working with.

Josh Williams, the captain, at Fire Station 14, B shift, reported early for duty and brought up the station and shift calendar on the office computer. "Hmm, the morning looks clear, have a crew meeting at 1400 at Station 10, and a ride along scheduled for 1700 to 2000, not a bad day," he thought to himself. The day was uneventful: Engine 14 made the meeting, ran a few calls, shopped for chow, and rolled into the station just before 1700 hours. As they were unpacking the groceries for the evening meal, the station doorbell rang.

"Hi, I'm Shelly Clark and this is my daughter Kindra. She's in eighth grade at Valley View Middle School and wanted to check out the fire department with me. There's a big eighth-grade dance tonight so we can't stay very long. I think Kindra wants to check things out and decide if she'll give me permission to test."

"Hello, Shelly. Hello Kindra," replied the firefighter answering the door. "I'm Rick, the senior firefighter here. Follow me and I'll introduce you to the captain and the rest of the crew." Things went real well, and after a brief station tour, Shelly went out to look at the truck and Kindra was helping the captain in the kitchen.

The station's dispatch lights came on and the dispatch followed, "Channel Six, 2 & 1 Assignment, house fire, across the street from 17244 Alamance Drive, Engine 14, Engine 17, Ladder 17, Battalion 2."

"Let's hit it! We're first due! This one's going to be working," yelled the captain as he headed to the apparatus bay. "Shelly you and Kindra sit in the middle, in the back where I showed you.

I don't want you getting off the truck until I come back and get you. Got it?"

They were both pretty wide-eyed at this point and only shook their heads up and down in compliance. The mother and daughter quickly buckled themselves in as the firefighters dressed in their protective gear. It was, in fact, a working fire as is usually the case when a fire is reported from across the street. The firefighters laid a supply line, took command, and started their initial fire attack and search.

After about an hour, the captain returned to the truck and leaned into the back to talk with Shelly and Kindra. "Sorry this took so long, it was in the attic so there was a lot of additional work to do. You guys can come out now. Put on these fire department safety vests and I'll show you what we did." As they stepped down from the rig, Shelly lightly grabbed the captain's arm and said, "I know you're busy but Kindra's really afraid that she'll miss the dance over at Valley View. Any idea about how much longer we'll be?"

"Well, let's see," the captain said as he looked over the scene. "We're almost finished here, probably only about 15 more minutes. Valley View is between here and Station 14. If it's OK with you we can drop her off and then take you to your car at the station."

"That's a great idea," Shelly answered. "I'll tell her. She'll be very relieved."

The captain showed them around the outside of the structure and explained to them what the fire investigator was doing and how the family was going to be assisted by the Red Cross. The crew finished loading the hose and placing all the hand tools back on the rig.

After 15 minutes, they were ready to take Kindra to her dance.

The crew and the "ride alongs" took their seats on the engine and they headed out of the neighborhood in the direction of Valley View Middle School. Upon arrival, the firefighter on Kindra's side jumped down from the rig and Kindra followed, jumping down and running toward the school gym.

Problem Solving

What Do You Know?

- Describe what you know about this incident.

What Do You Need to Know?

- What additional information would be helpful before further decision making?

Resources

- What potential resources would be helpful at this stage?

Responsibilities

- What legal, ethical, organizational, or interpersonal responsibilities should you consider?

Action Plan

- Decide what you would do next if you were in this situation.

Justification of Your Action Plan

- Explain the rationale you used for your decision.

Follow-up

- Would your action plan require any follow-up? Why or why not?

The Rest of the Story

Everything proceeded as planned. Shelly was safely delivered back to her car at Station 14. They all stood in the parking lot for a few minutes and Shelly thanked the crew, asked a few questions about the fire, and also wanted to know if she could come back for another ride. The crew was more than happy to invite her back and said that Kindra could come back too if she was not yet sure that she wanted her mother to be a firefighter. "Thank you all very much. This was very informative and I really appreciate your help in getting Kindra to her dance. Being a single mom can really be a challenge," Shelly stated as she got into her car.

The engine was further readied for the next call and the crew was entering the station for a little snack and a critique of the fire when the phone rang. "Captain Williams?" barked the B-shift battalion chief one.

"Yes, this is Josh," the captain replied. "What can I do for you?"

"You can take your truck out of service and wait in the quarters until the shift commander and I get there. Understand?"

"Well I'd like to know what's up but I understand," Josh replied. The only response he heard to that was a dial tone. He called the dispatch and informed them that Engine 14 would be out of service for an unknown time. He then went in and informed the crew of the phone call. They collectively shrugged their shoulders and wondered what it could be. The fire had gone well and nobody had got hurt. They'd just have to wait and see.

After about 25 minutes of sitting around in confusion and apprehension, the battalion chief and deputy chief finally arrived. They very seriously walked into the station and signaled Josh into the captain's office.

"What the hell were you doing with a teenaged girl on your rig? And why in the hell were you dropping her off at a dance at Valley View Middle School? This is scandalous and stupid. We thought you were smarter than this Josh," the battalion chief stormed as he marched around the office.

"Wait a minute chief, I can explain," pleaded Josh.

"You better explain and it better be good. We received multiple calls at Battalion Headquarters, the dispatch received a couple of calls, and one of those callers was a council member. We even had one lady request an officer to investigate and file a police report."

"Stop the presses chief. The girl's mother was on the rig with us and the explanation is very simple," Josh replied, trying to suppress a grin. After a lengthy explanation, the deputy chief and battalion chief were quite relieved and made a couple of quick phone calls to stop the frenzy. They also took Shelly's name and phone number in case anyone wanted to confirm the story.

As the chiefs were walking out of the station, they apologized to Josh and his crew for not having faith in them, and the battalion chief further explained, "You know guys this just goes to show you how important appearances are. I'm not saying that you did anything wrong, but I'm wondering how you could have handled this differently."

Discussion

- How could the Engine 14 captain and crew have handled this differently?
- Would a situation like this receive the same public reaction in your town or city?
- Has the public's trust of fire and emergency medical service (EMS) been eroded? If so, why?
- Are "ride alongs" a good idea or a bad idea?
- Does your agency have procedures in place about "ride alongs"? If so, what are they?

Skill Building

Public safety professionals are constantly subjected to public scrutiny. This is a fact of life in our avocations and is something we must all be very aware of and prepared for. Today's distrustful climate makes it necessary to review and plan for any and all contingencies. Had Captain Williams thought this through he may have asked Kindra's mother to also get off the rig, walk to the gym with Kindra, and report the situation to a school chaperone. Then, those observing would have seen a civilian adult with the teenaged girl. In some jurisdictions, this may have not appeared to be unusual. This is a great example of great customer service going wrong. Even though the intention was good, even good deeds must be thought through. The community's perception and relationship with their local emergency workers will have a great deal to do with how this would be perceived. However, we should never take our community's perception of us for granted. The reputation of your agency needs to be continually managed and built (Brunacini, 1996). Just because we see ourselves as the good guys does not mean that everyone else does.

As we are under continuous scrutiny, our actions receive a great deal of media attention. Those who work in emergency services are considered to be more than citizens; they are held to a higher standard. When one of our members breaks the law or does something contrary to acceptable community standards, they are singled out in the print, radio, and television media as Firefighter Smith or Paramedic Jones. We must all be aware that our actions on and off duty will be measured by a different yardstick, and we should act accordingly.

We build our relationship with the public by giving them access to us. We encourage people to drop by our quarters to see what we do and how we live. The public, for the most part, is interested in who we are and what we do. Our citizens want to know about our jobs; they respect what we do and build confidence in us through getting to know more about us, our equipment, and the way we live. Station/quarters tours and "ride alongs" are good things but must also be managed. Agencies should have some broad and basic guidelines on how station and quarters tours should be managed. For example, there is no place for unsupervised minors in a fire station or EMS quarters. All citizen observers should sign a document that records their age, contact information, etc. All citizen observers should also remain in the public areas of the station or quarters.

When determining whether our actions will be perceived by the public, it is a good idea to give them "the headline test." Ask yourself and each other, how would this look on the front page of tomorrow's paper: "Cinderella Dropped off at the Valley View Ball by Engine 14! No Glass Slipper and No Chaperone."

Lessons Learned

What Do You Know?

A mother and daughter came by Fire Station 14 for a tour and "ride along." During their visit, Engine 14 was dispatched to a working fire. The call took quite a while resulting in Kindra being late for a school dance. Rather than passing the school on the way back to the station, the mother agreed with the captain and they dropped Kindra off at the school. The trouble began when the mother did not get off the rig and escort her daughter into the dance. A member of the public, probably a parent of a child attending the dance, witnessed Kindra getting off the rig and running into the dance. Not knowing that Kindra's mother was on the truck, the parent reacted and acted in a manner that most good parents would: fear, disgust, and contempt. The parent took action and called the fire department to complain. The fire department administrators acted on the complaint.

What Do You Need to Know?

The facts are pretty straightforward and clear in this case. The most critical thing to recognize and know is that we are very much in the public eye. We are mostly viewed through a positive lens, but when all the information is not available, people will fill in the blanks, often from a negative and pessimistic point of view. Ride along and station tour standard operating procedures (SOPs) exist for a reason. It is extremely important for all crew members to become familiar with them.

Resources

Often, usually in haste, we sometimes do not think things through. This is especially true when in our personal perception we are doing nothing wrong. The most valuable resource to continuously check in with and utilize is a bit of skeptical common sense.

Responsibilities

The scene that played out did not break any laws and did not constitute a breach of ethics. The SOPs were followed; all necessary criteria were met and the proper forms completed. From the organizational perspective, some things could have been handled better. The supervisor must always have his or her radar on, monitoring the actions of his or her crew including where they go, what they are doing, and how they are acting; this information is then compared with any potential negative perceptions of those who are observing them in the public setting.

When evaluating what transpired from the interpersonal perspective, the battalion chief and deputy chief could have reacted in a more professional manner. In a perfect world, all supervisors should expect the best and prepare for the worst. It is wise to understand that a perception is just that. A perception is, at best, an imperfect view; all the facts are not present. If the facts were all known, it would be a reality, not a perception. Those we supervise should always be treated with respect, dignity, and forthright honesty.

Action Plan

In this scenario, most all that could have been done was done. The Engine 14 crew had to focus on accomplishing their mission and Kindra and her mother followed the instructions they were given. That said, it may have been a good practice for Captain Williams to check in with his riders when time allowed or ask that his engineer do it for him. If this had taken place, the fire department may have been able to secure the mother and daughter a ride back to the station, and this whole scenario and potential community relations problem could have been avoided.

However, this did occur, so the action plan must move to remediation and repair. Organizations will always experience the unexpected and should be prepared to deal with the occasional catastrophe as well as the occasional speed bump. Fortunately, what transpired in this case is a speed bump and can be easily handled with the lessons learned becoming part of the "ride along" knowledge base. The recommended steps to rectify this situation, appease the curious, and prevent future occurrences could include the following: The battalion chief calling the school principal during business hours and explaining how this was perceived and what actually happened. This action would provide the principal with information that could be utilized to answer questions should parents call. It may also be wise to ask the mother to call the school as well. Additionally, this scenario should be used as an educational tool to reinforce to all department members of the organization's visibility, and how critical it is to the mission to maintain a community standing.

Justification of Your Action Plan

This was not a tremendously serious situation providing that it was managed correctly after the fact. Disciplinary action need not take place. However, some steps would be required in an effort to inform those involved within both the department and the public. The action plan outlined in the previous section would appease those who thought the worst, informing them of the facts and avoiding any damaging rumors and innuendo.

Follow-up

The follow-up in this scenario would take place after the fact. After a reasonable amount of time had passed, it may be a good idea to call on the principal and find out if the school had received any phone calls or e-mails regarding the earlier incident. If not, all is well; if so, some further remediation may be required such as an open letter to all the parents with children at the school.

Summary

Alan Brunacini (Brunacini, 1996) states that fire department customer service can be evaluated around a number of guiding principles. One of those principals is to always be mindful of the way that what you are doing will look to other people. Even an act of good intention may be misinterpreted by those around us. Emergency responders should always be cognizant of how their behavior can be interpreted. For instance, is it a good practice to laugh and tell jokes at an emergency scene? How might the levity be interpreted by the victims, the family, the public, or the press? We ought to do our best to present ourselves in the most professional manner at all times. This may require us to go out of the way to explain what we are doing or the reasons we are doing something. The few minutes spent on this type of public relations will go a long way in preventing the type of misunderstandings such as the one in Glen Valley.

Chief Brunacini also states that we should regard everyone as a customer. This includes the citizens we serve, but also those who we work with. This is known as internal customer service. Good internal customer service works only in organizations that have good communication and a free flow of information. A third guiding principle is to always be nice and treat everyone with respect and dignity. For these principles to work, it is up to the senior officers to be the exemplars of these principles. When the senior management goes out of its way to provide good internal customer service, it will have positive effects throughout the organization. Good internal customer service will improve morale, increase pride in the organization, and encourage others to give good service to both the internal and external customers.

Key Terms

Ride Along   Structured programs in which citizens visit fire stations and ambulance quarters to get a better understanding of what we do and how we do it. This is a process many folks use to determine if they would like to work in our field and to also learn about the job in preparation for employment tests and job interviews.

References

Brunacini, A. (1996). *Essentials of Fire Department Customer Service.* Stillwater, OK: Fire Protection Publications.

A Quarter a Day Keeps the Doctor Away

Psychosocial, Ethical, and Leadership Dimensions

- EMS Protocols
- Interpersonal Skills
- Psychological Emergencies

226   **CASE STUDY 23:** *A Quarter a Day Keeps the Doctor Away*

A Quarter a Day Keeps the Doctor Away

Ladder 381 had just completed EMS training with its two probationary firefighters. The crew of five was just getting ready to sit down for lunch when the bell rang. "Ladder 381. Chest Pain. 7432 W. College Drive, in front of the library. Traffic on channel 6. Time out 1155." Lunch was going to have to wait. As the crew climbed into the truck, the senior paramedic thought that this would be an excellent opportunity for one of the new firefighters to practice the charting skills they had just reviewed. He told Firefighter Jones over the headset that he would be the one doing the charting on this call.

The only additional information from the dispatcher was that the patient was a 19-year-old male. This was not the typical chest pain patient. The two paramedics began reviewing all the different possibilities with the new firefighters. It could be a cardiac problem, but given his age, it could just as easily be anxiety or substance abuse.

The ladder made its way through the university campus and arrived at the library. Seated on a bench in front of the building was a college-aged male dressed in a T-shirt, cargo shorts, and a pair of flip-flops. The man was holding his arm across his stomach and began waving his cell phone at the truck as they pulled up. The captain approached the man while the crew grabbed the EMS gear off the truck.

"Did you call the fire department," asked the captain.

"Yes."

"Your chest is hurting you?"

"Yes."

"When did this start?

"About an hour ago."

"What's your name?"

"Chester."

"Alright Chester, we're going to examine you and get you fixed up."

By this time, the rest of the crew had walked up and were beginning the assessment. The captain informed them that the patient's name was Chester and that he had been experiencing chest pain for about an hour. One of the EMTs took vital signs. The engineer paramedic hooked Chester up to the cardiac monitor. The senior paramedic did a complete head to toe assessment and found no signs of trauma. Chester's vital signs were normal and the monitor showed normal sinus rhythm. As was typical of campus emergencies, a crowd of onlookers was beginning to gather. The captain did his best to keep them back until the campus police arrived to take over crowd control. The senior paramedic began to interview Chester.

"Chester, the monitor shows that your heart is beating normally. Your breathing and blood pressure are normal too. Can you tell me more about the chest pain you are having?"

"My heart is about to stop."

"Your heart is about to stop?"

"Yes, my heart is about to stop. Can I borrow fifteen cents?"

"What? . . . You say your heart is going to stop."

"That's right. I need fifteen cents," insisted Chester.

"Chester, do you know where you are right now?"

"Yeah, I'm at the college."

"And do you know what day it is?"

"Yes, it's Tuesday."

"That's right. And do you what year this is?"

"2006!"

"OK. Do you know who the president is?"

"Yeah, Cheney. Everybody knows that. Look, if you don't have fifteen cents, can I just have a nickel?"

"Chester, do you know why we are here?

"Yeah, I called you because my heart is going to stop."

By this time, both Chester and the medic were starting to get a little frustrated. Showing remarkable patience, the senior paramedic continued his interview.

"Chester, do you take any medications?"

"No, I stopped. If you don't have a nickel, I'll take pennies. I don't like to take pennies, but they will work if that's all you got."

"What medications were you taking Chester?"

"Zy...Zy...Zy....Zy-somethin'. I forget."

"Zyban?" interjected one of the new firefighters.

"No, that's not it," Chester replied. "Do any of you guys have any change?"

"Zyprexa?" queried the senior medic.

"That's it! I really need some change you guys."

"Chester, we don't have any change. Can you tell me where you live?"

"If you guys don't give me some change fast, my heart is going to stop!"

Problem Solving

What Do You Know?

- Describe what you know about this incident.

What Do You Need to Know?

- What additional information would be helpful before further decision making?

Resources

- What potential resources would be helpful at this stage?

Responsibilities

- What legal, ethical, organizational, or interpersonal responsibilities should you consider?

Action Plan

- Decide what you would do next if you were in this situation.

Justification of Your Action Plan

- Explain the rationale you used for your decision.

Follow-up

* Would your action require any follow-up? Why or why not?

The Rest of the Story

As they continued to talk for 20 minutes, the senior paramedic finally got Chester to reveal his belief that he needed to swallow at least 25 cents a day to pay for his heart to beat. Because he had swallowed only a dime that day, he was becoming anxious that his heart would stop. The campus police learned from one of the students in the crowd that Chester had been panhandling in front of the library for more than a week. Chester carried no identification. He either could not remember where he lived or was choosing not to disclose this information. The medics contacted the base hospital and transported him there for further evaluation.

At the hospital, it was learned that Chester had been a student at the university the previous semester. He had been treated at the university counseling center and had received his medication from student health services. He had failed to complete any of his classes and did not continue as a student. Since he was no longer a student, he was no longer eligible to receive mental health services from the university. Chester's roommates had recently thrown him out because they had grown tired of his bizarre behavior and because he was consistently stealing change from their rooms.

Discussion

* What did the crew in this scenario do right?
* Did the crew do anything wrong?
* Do you think Chester presented a danger to himself or others?
* Do you think that patients with mental illness are given the same level of respect that medical patients receive? Explain your answer.

Skill Building

Chester's belief that he had to swallow coins to pay for his heart to beat is an example of delusional thinking. Delusions are beliefs that are maintained even in light of convincing evidence or arguments that they are false. Delusions are characteristic of a psychotic disorder. Psychotic disorders represent a condition distinguished by a severe mental break with reality. It is not uncommon for individuals to experience their first such break in young adulthood (Comer, 2007).

Chester's thinking manifested itself in the bizarre behavior of swallowing coins. This behavior is an example of the disorder pica. Pica is a rare condition in which patients compulsively eat things not normally consumed as food. Although coin swallowing by adults is not something that is commonly encountered, it should be considered a behavior that is a danger to self (Comer, 2007).

Coins can get lodged as they pass through the body. In children, this can sometimes lead to a choking episode. In Chester's case, the number of coins he was swallowing could prevent him from being able to clear his bowels as they accumulate in his digestive track. Research conducted at Duke University has shown that the chemical reaction between the zinc found in pennies and stomach acid is similar to that in wet cell batteries and is caustic to the stomach lining (O'Hara et al., 1999).

Chester was being treated with Zyprexa. Zyprexa is the brand name for the atypical antipsychotic medication olanzapine. Zyprexa is a tablet usually taken orally once daily. Its side effects include high fever, tachycardia, excessive perspiration, and muscle rigidity. In rare cases, it can cause seizures. An overdose of Zyprexa will usually be characterized by slurred speech and excessive sedation (Thomas & Woodall, 2006).

The medication Zyban was also mentioned in this case. Zyban is a brand name for the antidepressant medication bupropion. It is prescribed for tobacco cessation. Zyban is a 150-mg tablet taken twice daily. It works at the neurological level to reduce cravings for nicotine. Its side effects include anxiety, insomnia, restlessness, dry mouth, constipation, and appetite suppression. Less frequently encountered side effects include nausea, dizziness, severe headache, confusion, cardiac arrhythmia, and seizures. Overdose symptoms are confusion, agitation, seizures, and coma (Thomas & Woodall, 2006).

This case is a good example of how taking the time to do a good interview can help to determine the real cause of a problem. This could have been accomplished faster had the medic simply engaged Chester in a mental status exam. This crew could have easily determined that there was nothing medically wrong with Chester and asked him to sign a release. To their credit, they spent a considerable amount of time with Chester and were able to identify his psychotic condition. They realized his self-destructive behavior and transported him to the hospital for further evaluation.

This crew could have improved their encounter with Chester by doing a few simple things. The captain asked Chester his name but he never introduced himself. The senior paramedic did not introduce himself either. Emergency responders should always introduce themselves by telling the patient their name, their job title, and their agency affiliation. If it is appropriate, they may also want to display their credentials (Thomas & Woodall, 2006). We cannot assume that because we arrive in emergency vehicles and we are wearing uniforms that every patient understands who we are and why we are there. In addition, EMS providers should always ask permission before they start assessing a patient. Some people may have a strong reaction to being touched by a stranger. This reaction could be the result of gender or cultural differences, a history of abuse or domestic violence, medical conditions, mental illness, substance abuse, etc.

This crew treated Chester with respect and dignity. They refrained from making judgments about his condition and displayed a calm, caring, and compassionate attitude. Most emergency medical service (EMS) providers receive extensive training in treating medical emergencies.

The same cannot be said for treating psychological emergencies. When combined with the fact that the majority of EMS calls are for medical emergencies, EMS providers also have fewer opportunities to develop the skills to effectively work with mentally ill patients. In fact, some EMS providers may not consider treating and caring for those suffering from mental illness as part of their job. Patient care could be improved by increasing the number of hours spent training for psychological emergencies and including scenario-based encounters with mentally ill patients.

Lessons Learned

What Do You Know?

Ladder 381 was dispatched to the university library for someone experiencing chest pain. The dispatcher was able to tell them that the patient was a 19-year-old male. The medics reviewed all the possibilities while en route. When they arrived on scene, they found the patient sitting on a bench in front of the library. The patient informed them that he had been experiencing chest pain for the past hour. The crew examined him and found that his vital signs and electrocardiogram (EKG) were normal. One of the paramedics interviewed the patient and determined that he was alert and oriented. During the course of the interview, the patient kept asking to borrow 15 cents. The crew ignored his request and the medic continued the interview. The medic determined that the patient was previously taking Zyprexa but that he had stopped. Eventually, the patient stated that his heart was going to stop if the crew did not give him some spare change.

The medic interviewed the patient for 20 minutes and discovered that the patient believed he needed to swallow 25 cents each day to pay for his heart to beat. The patient was transported to the hospital where it was learned that he had been receiving mental health services at the university. Since he did not continue as a student, the university was not able to continue his treatment. Additionally, the patient's roommates had kicked him out and he did not have a place to live.

What Do You Need to Know?

The successful outcome of this call was predicated on the fact that the paramedic knew how to conduct a brief mental status exam. This ability ought to be part of every EMS provider's skill set.

Resources

It is a good idea to request assistance from law enforcement any time there is the potential for an EMS incident to attract a crowd. Not having to worry about crowd control allows the EMS professionals to focus on patient care. In this case, the campus police were able to obtain some information about the patient from the other students who had gathered. This illustrates the fact that onlookers can also be a resource. Sometimes a simple question such as "Did anyone see what happened?" can yield valuable information.

Responsibilities

EMS responders have the obligation to assess and treat a patient's condition. Assessing a psychological condition is not straightforward and frequently takes more time than it does to assess medical problems.

Action Plan

The actions taken by this crew were correct. Once they determined that the patient was suffering from a mental illness, they transported him to the emergency department. Hopefully, this began a chain of events and referrals that would allow the patient to get the treatment he needed. This was especially pertinent in this case because the patient was no longer eligible to receive services from the university's health center.

Justification of Your Action Plan

The crew in this case recognized that the behavior of swallowing coins represented a danger to self. EMS protocols mandate transport to the hospital.

Follow-up

In this case, the crew did everything they should have. Other than documenting the call, no other follow-up is necessary.

Summary

Although it is not the role of EMS providers to diagnose and treat mental illness, EMS providers should be able to assess and report psychological symptoms. Reporting the symptoms accurately will help the physician to formulate a treatment plan. Psychological symptoms can easily be identified by learning a few simple assessments. The first is a brief mental status exam. The brief mental status exam provides information about a patient's orientation, physical appearance, speech, and body language. A full mental status exam will yield additional information regarding affect or mood, cognition, thought content, and judgment.

The brief psychosocial history can be used to give us a more in-depth look at a patient's level of functioning. In addition to the history of the presenting problem, it includes information concerning the patient's psychological history and his or her current level of functioning. The assessment of functioning includes activities of daily living, home life, work and/or school, leisure time, and stress management skills. The full psychosocial history takes account of a patient's emotional and behavioral history.

Equally important is the ability to do a lethality assessment. A lethality assessment allows us to determine if a person is a danger to themselves or others. Sadly, we must also have the ability to determine if patients have been the victim of violence. We must be skilled at recognizing the signs of child abuse, elder abuse, the abuse of a dependent adult, domestic violence, and sexual assault.

A key factor in the ability to do these types of assessments is strong interpersonal skills. In conducting a good assessment, we must ask questions of a highly personal or sensitive nature. If patients are uncomfortable, they may be reluctant to answer truthfully. The ability to put patients at ease and to make them feel safe, comfortable, and cared for is a crucial skill for any EMS provider.

Key Terms

Anxiety   A vague, unpleasant emotional state with the qualities of apprehension, dread, distress, and uneasiness.

Delusions   A belief that is maintained in spite of argument, data, and refutation that should (reasonably) be sufficient to destroy it.

Mental Status Exam   A full clinical work-up of a psychiatric patient including the assessment of overall psychiatric condition, diagnosis of existing disorders, prognosis, estimates of suitability for treatment of various kinds, formulation of overall personality, and compilation of historical and developmental data.

Pica   A rare condition in which patients compulsively eat things not normally consumed as food.

Psychotic Condition   Referring to the total mental condition of a person who has suffered a break from reality at a specific moment.

Psychotic Disorder   Often used to describe a set of symptoms characterized by delusional thinking and/or hallucinations.

Zyban   The brand name for the antidepressant medication bupropion. It is prescribed for tobacco cessation.

Zyprexa   The brand name for the atypical antipsychotic medication olanzapine.

References

Comer, R. J. (2007). *Abnormal Psychology*, 6th edition. New York, NY: Worth Publishers.

O'Hara, S. M., Donnelly, L. F., Chuang, E., Briner, W. H., & Bisset III, G. S. (1999). The Radiographic Appearance and Hazards of Gastric Retention of Zinc-Based Pennies. *Radiology* 213, 113–17.

Thomas, J., & Woodall, S. J. (2006). *Responding to Psychological Emergencies: A Field Guide*. Clifton Park, NY: Thomson-Delmar Learning.

Professional Courtesy?

Psychosocial, Ethical, and Leadership Dimensions

- EMS Protocols
- Interagency Cooperation
- Patient Advocacy
- Standard Operating Procedures
- Team Dynamics

Professional Courtesy?

Corry had been working as much overtime as he could get in hopes of having enough money to finish the addition on his house. It wasn't too bad because he loved his job as an EMT with the South County Ambulance Company. He'd been working there since he completed his EMT certification some six years ago. He had developed into a highly respected EMT and had even pursued additional training in farm emergencies and farm rescue.

Earlier in the evening, Corry had just completed another 16 hours of overtime and felt that he deserved a little rest and relaxation. As he was driving north on County Road 5, he decided to stop for a few beers at the Ole' Brass Rail, a favorite cop, fire, and EMS watering hole. He had changed out of his uniform before he left the ambulance head-quarters, so he was ready to have some fun. As he made his way from the door to the bar, he spotted many familiar faces. One thing he liked about working in a small town was that everybody knew everybody. He'd lived here since his first year of high school and was pretty sure he'd never leave. One beer led to another and another, Corry was hav-ing so much fun with his friends that he neglected to eat, and several hours later, it was dark out and he was drunk.

South County Ambulance 54 arrived on the scene just in front of the Blue Springs Volunteer Fire Company. Three county sheriff's cars were already on the scene. The call had come in as a single vehicle in a ditch, which was common on these narrow country roads. Jill re-ported "on scene" and looked up to see a familiar deputy headed her way. "Hey Jill, we've got a single car in the ditch. The air bag deployed but the guy says he's not injured and doesn't appear to be."

"Thanks Dirk, we'll take a look," replied Jill as she patted him on the shoulder.

"Ah, just a second Jill, you might not want to go over there just yet," Dirk said grabbing Jill's arm.

"What do ya mean Dirk?" she replied.

"Well, it's Corry and he appears to be pretty drunk," was the deputy's reply.

Problem Solving

What Do You Know?

- Describe what you know about this incident.

What Do You Need to Know?

- What additional information would be helpful before further decision making?

Resources

- What potential resources would be helpful at this stage?

Responsibilities

- What legal, ethical, organizational, or interpersonal responsibilities should you consider?

Action Plan

- Decide what you would do next if you were in this situation.

Justification of Your Action Plan

- Explain the rationale you used for your decision.

Follow-up

- Would your action plan require any follow-up? Why or why not?

The Rest of the Story

"Oh crap! This is just great! You know he'll lose his job if he loses his license," Jill said shaking her head.

"Well Jill, Corry and I go way back. I've talked to Ned and Buck and they're OK with having the car towed and taking him home."

Jill held up her hand as if to say stop, "Dirk, I've got to check him out. What if he's got an internal bleed or a head injury? If we take him home and he dies or is forced to go in later, we'd all be in a heck of a jam."

"It's your call Jill but if you go over there and make contact with him, all bets are off. If you examine him, the paper trail will be started and we'll have to do what we have to do on our end," Dirk said shrugging his shoulders.

Discussion

- What happens if Jill and her partner make patient contact with Corry?
- What could happen legally if Jill did not make patient contact with Corry?
- What position should the volunteer firefighters take on this?
- Is this an example of ethical behavior on the part of the sheriff's department?
- Is this an example of "professional courtesy" going too far?
- Is this something that we can expect to happen only in the rural environment?

Skill Building

What to do? There has been a dispatch, a wreck, and a driver, and the results have been witnessed by three different agencies and their personnel. Corry is a well-liked and respected friend and fellow employee of several folks on the scene. No one wants to see Corry suffer and probably even lose his job. If the emergency responders attempt to alter what has happened, breaching policy and protocol, a series of events could ensue. If Jill and her partner elect not to chart Corry, they are in serious breach of EMS protocols and may even be guilty of patient abandonment. This could lead to severe disciplinary action, up to and including termination and/or legal ramifications against Jill and her partner. Furthermore, they could be placing Corry's life in jeopardy. If they chose to chart Corry, it would be necessary to document that the patient had consumed an unknown quantity of alcohol. Needless to say, driving under the influence (DUI) and driving while intoxicated (DWI) are crimes. The sheriffs would then be forced to act, performing the tasks that the law requires them to perform.

The volunteer firefighters are also witnesses to this call. They were not consulted on their feelings regarding this situation, but their positions and certifications would also be placed at risk should the sheriff just take Corry home.

Those serving the public are held to a higher community standard. As public safety professionals, EMS and fire personnel should hold themselves to a higher standard as well as exercise personal responsibility for their on- and off-duty actions and behaviors. A final critical question should be: Would Corry want to assume the responsibility of placing his friends' and colleagues' jobs at risk?

Lessons Learned

What Do You Know?

We know that there has been a single vehicle accident in which the driver is a respected, local EMT. The county sheriff's officers and the local volunteer fire department are already on the scene when the ambulance company arrives. The deputies are willing to tow the car and take the driver home. However, all parties agree that if the EMS crew examines and charts him, then the probable DUI/DWI will have to be documented and Corry will eventually be charged and possibly convicted. As the scenario ends, a decision as to whether to treat and document has not been made.

What Do You Need to Know?

It would be nice to know if Corry was going to be OK but that's not possible unless he is assessed, treated, and possibly transported for even further diagnosis and treatment. The impact, in this case, was severe enough for the air bag to deploy, so the injuries may be serious. It is also imperative to know and understand your agency's standard operating procedures (SOPs), EMS protocols, and your state's DUI laws.

Resources

The resources necessary to serve the victim are all on the scene. The question is, Will all the required resources be utilized as required by the law, EMS protocols, SOPs, and ethical considerations? Of course higher-level supervision could be called to the scene, which would take the decision out of the hands of those on the scene but would more than likely result in Corry being assessed, treated, and transported for further evaluation.

Responsibilities

Each and every public safety agency has a legal and ethical responsibility to perform its respective duties according to the law, their protocols, and their SOPs. In this scenario, the sheriff's deputies were willing to ignore all their responsibilities in the interest of helping a friend. The question remains, What were Jill and her partner going to do? They held a serious responsibility on several levels. How they decided to fulfill that responsibility would have life-changing ramifications to either one person or potentially many. We must follow EMS protocols, SOPs, and laws. Failing to do so is a violation of public trust.

Action Plan

The advisable action plan in this case would be to assess, treat, document, and possibly transport Corry. The risks of not fulfilling their responsibilities are simply too great. Their documentation would have to include their findings of ethyl alcohol (EtOH) onboard the patient. When it was determined that Corry was going to be treated at the scene, Jill and her partner should probably call a supervisor. It is better to involve higher-level supervisors sooner than later. The ambulance company's administrative staff would be best prepared to document this case, gather available evidence, and initiate the evaluation process from a personnel perspective.

Justification of Your Action Plan

All action plans must be based on the agency's SOPs and grounded in the legal, ethical, and morale considerations. The ramifications of electing to ignore these responsibilities are simply too great for Corry, for Jill and her partner, and for the sheriff's deputies on the scene.

Follow-up

Follow-up in this scenario would require that Corry's fellow responders and administrators make themselves available to help him heal from his injuries, maneuver the legal system, and work through any personnel action. Corry may feel angry and abandoned and visible support would be the best possible way to help him get through this situation, pay the price, and perhaps move on.

Summary

Altering the facts in this situation constitutes a "cover-up," so this would be not only an unethical breach of duty on the part of the sheriff's department but also a crime. Professional courtesy (as those within the business refer to it) does exist and is not always a bad thing. However, in this case, what these deputies are willing to do for Corry is an example of going too far. Professional courtesy is extended in both rural and city environments. It is an informal process that is quietly accepted, rarely talked about, and when extended, never spoken of to the general public. It is not necessarily expected but always appreciated when extended. We must always ask ourselves, Where do we draw the line? Actions such as those proposed in this case study could lead to further cover-ups and could also perpetuate a dangerous cycle in the form of: "Well we did this for you and it's now time to return the favor."

Key Terms

DUI   Under this condition, the legal blood/alcohol limits are defined on a state-by-state basis.

DWI   Under this condition, the legal blood/alcohol limits are defined on a state-by-state basis.

EtOH   It is found in alcoholic beverages. This designation is frequently used in the emergency medical and law enforcement field setting to describe and document a person under the influence of alcohol.

Professional Accountability   The set of accountability standards employers hold to employees. Employees also hold a share in holding themselves professional accountable.

Professional Courtesy   An informal process in which law enforcement extends greater latitude to a fellow officer, EMS personnel, firefighters, and other public officials.

Personal Responsibility   The set of personal standards that an individual holds to himself or herself. Personal responsibility is driven by the person's belief system, world view, work ethic, and morals.

Mechanism of Injury   The process of examining evidence available on the scene in an effort to better determine and assign a triage level to a patient impacted by the mechanism. This is not an exact science, but it is often utilized in cases involving patients in motor vehicle accidents. The mechanism of injury often leads to the upgrading of the medical level assigned to a patient in cases where the damage to the mechanism is severe.

Frequent Flyer

Psychosocial, Ethical, and Leadership Dimensions

- Compassion Fatigue
- Customer Service
- Health and Wellness
- Interagency Cooperation
- Team Dynamics

Frequent Flyer

Ernie had smoked heavily for over 30 years. He had also bravely served his country in World War II. But in the last few years of his life, time and smoking had caught up with him, leaving him constantly in respiratory distress. The sucking sounds from his stoma could be heard in the next room. Ernie was miserable, and in his mind, there was no relief in sight.

In his frustration, Ernie would moan and carry on until his family had no choice but to call 9-1-1. The various ambulance and fire/EMS agencies that responded knew Ernie well, and as dispatch read the address, everyone on duty knew that Ernie was calling again. His frequent calls for service were becoming very frustrating to the responders and his family. Many times he was transported twice a day: once in the morning and again late at night. The hospital, adhering to the latest managed care philosophy and knowing that there was little that they could do, would simply evaluate him, check his oxygen saturation levels, and then release him. This frustrating cycle continued on for what seemed to be an eternity. Upon arrival, most crews would crank up his home oxygen and change him from a nasal cannula to a mask over the stoma at 15 liters-per-minute.

These actions rarely pacified Ernie. He would cover his stoma, and in his raspy-wheezy voice say, "I wanna go to the hospital. Take me to the VA." His veteran's benefits would cover the VA but that hospital was some 25 miles away and there were at least three closer hospitals. As the cycle continued, the attitudes of the responders degraded into frustration, anger, and resentment.

"There's nothing we can do for this guy. How can he get away with abusing the system?"

"I hate running on Ernie. His sheets always smell like piss. Why doesn't his family take better care of him?"

Common questions at shift change were "Did you run on Ernie yesterday? Did you transport him? What time of day was it?" If the answer was yes, the response was always "Good, maybe we'll be off the hook today." Running on Ernie became so frustrating that crews actually dreaded the call. Once in the middle of the night, the engine was dispatched to Ernie's. When the call came in, the captain sat up in bed and stated, "I'm not running on Ernie again! You guys go without me!" The crew responded a person short as they had little choice. The captain later claimed that he was talking in his sleep, but the crew had their doubts.

Problem Solving

What Do You Know?

- Describe what you know about this incident.

What Do You Need to Know?

- What additional information is required before further decision making?

Resources

- What potential resources would be helpful at this stage?

Responsibilities

- What legal, ethical, organizational, or interpersonal responsibilities should you consider?

Action Plan

- Decide what you would do next if you were in this situation.

Justification of Your Action Plan

- Explain the rationale you used for your decision.

Follow-up

- Would your action plan require any follow-up? Why or why not?

The Rest of the Story

Some ambulance and fire department crews would honor his wishes and take Ernie to the VA hospital, while others would insist that he go to the closest facility for evaluation and treatment. Other crews, depending on the time of day or night, would attempt to convince him that all that could be done for him was being done for him at home and that no hospital transport was needed. After about 2 years of Ernie constantly calling 9-1-1, the cycle came to an end. Ernie passed away.

Discussion

- Do you think Ernie's behavior represented an abuse of the local emergency medical service (EMS) system?
- Should those in need (real or perceived) be limited in the number of times they can call for help?
- Was it ethical to take Ernie to the closest appropriate facility even those times he was stable enough to go to the hospital of his choosing?
- Do services exist that might have been able to assist with Ernie's care in your area? If so, what are they and how can they be accessed?
- How can the negative attitudes toward patients such as Ernie be prevented?

Skill Building

In this scenario, Ernie's breathing problem frustrated him and had his family to their wits' end. They probably felt that they had no one else to turn to and no other resources from which to draw assistance. The EMS system and the hospital were their only hope. Did this constitute system abuse? No. This was a family and a patient attempting to access the healthcare system in the only way they knew: by dialing 9-1-1. It would be ludicrous to limit the number of times a family can call 9-1-1 for assistance. However, it may have been possible to create a better situation for all involved through discussions and planning with the family, the Veterans Administration (VA) hospital case manager, and even local social service agencies. As is true with most challenges, you can't take the same actions over and over again and expect a different outcome.

All EMS responders have a set of regional and national protocols that must be adhered to. In general terms, one of those mandates is the patient's right to choose the hospital they want to be transported to, providing that their condition is stable. The ambulance and fire crews were taking the path of least resistance if their medical assessment demonstrated that Ernie was stable enough to make the longer trip to the VA hospital. Their actions may not have been unethical, since they were, in fact, transferring Ernie to a higher medical authority, but what did their actions provide in the way of a long-term solution to the problem?

These types of calls are frustrating and do take a toll on crew morale. Management should seek ways to validate the feelings and reactions of these responders. This is not about crews being lazy or not wanting to do their job. Calls of this type need to be placed on the agendas of crew meetings and officers meetings. Alternative and creative remedies should be sought. The local social services agencies or the VA hospital may have had some care and transportation programs that could have provided home care and alternative transportation options.

The EMS responder should be aware, in advance, that patients like Ernie come with the territory. The EMS system is a component of the larger healthcare system. The larger health system does not distinguish between what is an emergency and what is not. Again, that determination belongs to the caller. It can, at times, be necessary to reframe our personal expectations of what our job is and what our mission entails. Basically, it is to serve those who call no matter what they call for and whenever they call and to serve them to the best of our individual and collective abilities.

Lessons Learned

What Do You Know?

Ernie was a senior citizen and a veteran who was suffering from chronic obstructive pulmonary disease (COPD) brought on from many years of smoking. The quality of Ernie's health slowly deteriorated as it became harder and harder for him to breathe, which is the characteristic of this disease. In frustration over his inability to catch his breath, Ernie would carry on and demand to be taken to the hospital. As there is no cure for COPD, there was not much that could be done.

As his condition worsened, Ernie and his family got to the point where they were calling 9-1-1 for EMS almost every day. Although there were closer hospitals, Ernie always insisted on being transported to the VA hospital for his care. This began to take a toll on the responders to the point that they became frustrated and started to resent Ernie's call for service.

What Do You Need to Know?

EMS must respond to every call for service. Difficulty breathing always results in the dispatch of advanced life support (ALS) units. EMS protocols dictate that patients with difficulty breathing be transported to the emergency department.

Resources

Some communities may have other options for the transport of patients like Ernie. These resources may be located in various social service agencies. Every community is served by an Area Agency on Aging. These agencies are part of a national network of organizations that were established under the Older Americans Act of 1971 (State of Oregon, 2006). Ernie may have also had a case manager at the VA hospital.

Responsibilities

We are obligated to respond to patients each and every time they call for service. This responsibility does not change based on the number of times they have requested service. EMS providers and their management have the responsibility to monitor themselves, their coworkers, and their employees for signs of burnout and compassion fatigue. If these signs become evident, employees have the responsibility for self-care and should seek professional help if needed. Management has the responsibility to provide resources for self-care and access to professional services.

Action Plan

We must respond to Ernie and transport him to the VA hospital, whenever it is determined that he is stable enough to make the trip.

Justification of Your Action Plan

EMS protocols obligate us to transport every patient who has difficulty breathing. Patients have the right to choose the hospital at which they will receive care. We are obligated to honor their choice of hospital except in the event of life-threatening emergency or when they sign a refusal of transport.

Follow-up

EMS responders may want to consider connecting Ernie to the other resources available to him. After responding to Ernie, responders may want to consider a brief defusing where they can talk openly about their feelings and frustrations. They may also want to contact Ernie's case worker at the VA hospital regarding his treatment plan or potential changes to that plan.

Summary

The behavior of the EMS responders in this case exhibits the frustration that is experienced when we feel powerless or unable to help a patient. Most EMS responders have a strong desire to provide care and help for the sick and injured. Being able to do this is a tremendous source of gratification for doing a difficult job. In this case, there was nothing that could be done for Ernie. The fact that they were unable to help contributed to their feelings of resentment.

The EMS providers at this agency failed to recognize that they were experiencing the symptoms of compassion fatigue and burnout.

Likewise, their supervisors and management team also failed to recognize the signs. When employees don't like coming to work, or don't like performing their essential job functions, the morale of an agency will quickly decline. The fact that this occurred over a 2-year period represents an almost complete breakdown of the team dynamics and the management system of this agency.

This type of breakdown almost always results in poor job performance and poor customer service. It is highly likely that the resentment these responders felt showed in their attitude when treating Ernie. It is likely that they became complacent and sluggish. They probably expected each call to be just like the last. When this happens, we run the risk of hurrying through our assessments and may miss subtle changes or key findings. Clearly, these responders lost sight of their role as patient advocates.

Several things could have been done from an organizational perspective to alleviate what was happening. Management could have recognized the signs of burnout in their employees and taken steps to intervene. They could have partnered with other agencies to find other solutions for Ernie. They could have held debriefings and let their employees express their feelings. They could have utilized an employee assistance program (EAP) to help those who need more support. If possible, they could have made changes in staffing patterns to give employees a break from responding to Ernie. It may have also been possible to look at dispatch and deployment strategies and increase the number of different units that responded to Ernie.

Key Terms

Compassion Fatigue   Commonly referred to as "burnout"; this term describes individuals usually working in the helping professions who have, for various reasons, lost their ability to effectively manage their personal and professional relationships with work team members, family members, supervisors, and those they serve.

This is frequently caused by being overworked, continual exposure to the negative aspects of the human condition, and fatigue including sleep deprivation.

Defusing   The term given to the process of talking something through.

Employee Assistance Program   A benefit program provided by the employer that usually offers assessment, short-term counseling, and referral services.

Managed Care   A model in the U.S. healthcare delivery that is intended to reduce unnecessary healthcare costs.

Morale   The capacity of people to maintain belief in an institution, in a goal, or even in oneself and others.

Healthcare System   The organization and the method by which health care is provided.

Social Services   Agencies concerned with the causes, solutions, and human impacts of social problems.

References

State of Oregon (2006). *History of the Older Americans Act.* Salem, OR: State of Oregon Department of Human Services.

This Is My Patient

Psychosocial, Ethical, and Leadership Dimensions

- Diversity
- EMS Protocols
- Interagency Cooperation
- Standard Operating Procedures
- Safety
- Team Dynamics

▓▓▓▓▓▓ **This Is My Patient**

Fire Station 3 is located in a small suburb mostly populated by retirees. As part of their mutual aid agreement, they also respond to the neighboring Native American reservation. Such was the case when Engine 3 was dispatched to an unconscious party at a private residence on the reservation. When they arrived, they found a middle-aged Native American male lying face down in the front yard. As they pulled the gear off the truck, an elderly man emerged from the house and began yelling at them in his native language. As the two paramedics moved to treat the patient, the captain attempted to reassure the elderly gentleman that they were there to help.

The two medics and the EMT quickly realized that the man was in full code and began resuscitation efforts. The captain met with little success in his efforts to calm the elderly gentleman because of the obvious language barrier. The rest of the crew had started CPR and were preparing to defibrillate the patient. At this time, an ambulance from the reservation arrived with two Native American paramedics. One medic went to assist the captain, while the other joined the resuscitation efforts. The elderly gentleman continued his tirade and began speaking with the Native American medic from the ambulance. After this brief interchange, the elderly man went back inside his house.

The two medics from the ambulance told the crew from Engine 3 that they could take it from here and that they should leave. The captain balked at this suggestion explaining that he was in command of this scene and that every person here was needed to properly work the code. The medics repeated their request with an increased sense of urgency. They explained that the elderly gentleman was the patient's father and that he was not comfortable letting his son be treated by the three Caucasian men and one Caucasian woman who were working on Engine 3 that day. The captain remained steadfast that his crew would remain on scene and continue to treat the patient.

Problem Solving

What Do You Know?

- Describe what you know about this incident.

What Do You Need to Know?

- What additional information is required before further decision making?

Resources

- What potential resources would be helpful at this stage?

Responsibilities

- What legal, ethical, organizational, or interpersonal responsibilities should you consider?

Action Plan

- Decide what you would do next if you were in this situation.

Justification of Your Action Plan

- Explain the rationale you used for your decision.

Follow-up

- Would your action plan require any follow-up? Why or why not?

The Rest of the Story

After a minute, the elderly man reemerged from the house with a shotgun and resumed his tirade. The two medics from the ambulance looked at the captain and again advised him to leave. Sensing that his crew might be in danger, the captain ordered his crew back to the truck. They made a hasty retreat as the two ambulance medics continued to work the patient and the elderly gentleman continued shouting and waving his shotgun.

Discussion

- Do you agree with the captain's decision to leave the scene? Why or why not?
- Did the Engine 3 crew violate any standard emergency medical service (EMS) protocols?
- Did the ambulance paramedics violate any standard EMS protocols?
- How will you respond to an individual who does not speak the same language as you do?
- Suggest some other strategies that this captain could have used in this situation.

Skill Building

Many times our customers are from different cultures and ways of life from our own. If we work in an area where we know that we will be encountering people from different cultures, it is incumbent upon us to familiarize ourselves with that culture and to respect their wishes. It is true even when those wishes are at odds with our agency's protocols and procedures. It doesn't mean that we must necessarily learn their language, but it does mean that we should have a working familiarization with the customs and ways of those we may be serving. If there are different cultures and subcultures within the potential response area of our agency, it would be wise to seek leaders and resources within that community and start a healthy dialogue.

Without a working knowledge of the cultures you may be responding in, you might also be placing yourself and those you are responsible for at risk. This case study serves as an example of just how things can negatively escalate when neither the responder nor the recipient of the service understand each other. This was more than a language barrier. This was a case in which a little knowledge about cultural differences could have helped to avoid a less than desirable outcome.

The lack of understanding also led to a potential standard of care compromise. Fortunately, the two tribal EMS responders were paramedics. Therefore, when the captain opted to leave the scene, he passed the patient from one ALS crew to another ALS crew. The compromise of the standard of care became an issue of adequate personnel, not an issue of abandonment. Leaving the scene also mitigated a situation that could have easily escalated to violence. The safety of EMS responders always needs to take precedence over treatment. Had the captain insisted on staying, he would have been placing his crew in a dangerous situation. If the ambulance had not arrived, the captain may have had to request assistance from the tribal police department and moved to a staging location until the scene was secure.

When examining the interagency and organizational issues, some definite considerations come to mind. A mutual assistance/mutual aid contract represents much more than establishing an operational plan. This type of agreement invites folks working for another community into other jurisdictions and asks them to effectively manage and mitigate a given set of very tragic and traumatic circumstances. In most cases, these communities are pretty homogenous. However, in some instances cultures, customs and language are markedly different. When this is true, some serious consideration, planning, and even special training are in order.

Lessons Learned

What Do You Know?

Because of a mutual/automatic aid agreement, Engine 3 responded out of their jurisdiction to the neighboring reservation. When they arrived, they found a middle-aged Native American male in full arrest. They were also met by an elderly Native American man who was agitated and shouting at them in a language they did not understand. The crew worked the code while the captain tried to reassure and calm down the elderly gentleman.

Shortly thereafter, two Native American paramedics arrived on an ambulance from the reservation. One of the medics assisted the crew, while the other spoke with the elderly gentleman. After talking with the gentleman, the medic told the captain that he and his partner would take it from here and that the engine crew should leave because the man's father did not want Caucasians treating his son. The captain refused to leave because it would violate EMS protocols and standard operating procedures. The gentleman reemerged from the house with a shotgun. Seeing this, the captain changed his mind and left with his crew.

What Do You Need to Know?

Every EMS provider needs to understand the EMS protocols in their system and the standard operating procedures of their agency. This case gives an example of why it is important to have knowledge of beliefs and customs found in all the different cultures that may be represented in you response area.

Resources

In this case, part of the problem was cultural and part of the problem was the language barrier. Anytime we meet a citizen whom we are unable to communicate with, it may be wise to call for an interpreter. In larger metropolitan areas, an interpreter may be able to respond to the scene, but this may not be the case in smaller or more isolated communities. A number of companies are able to provide interpreter service via telephone or cell phone.

Responsibilities

EMS protocols and standard operating procedures dictate our responsibilities for patient care. It is important to remember that our safety must come before patient care.

Action Plan

In this case, the captain made the correct decision. If an ambulance from the reservation had not come, the crew may still have had to leave the scene and leave the patient behind. In that case, they would have to stage a safe distance from the scene and request assistance from law enforcement.

Justification of Your Action Plan

Leaving the scene is the only decision when being threatened with a weapon or with harm, and law enforcement is not present. The captain was unable to communicate with the patient's father and was unable to calm him down. There is no justifiable reason to put yourself or your crew in harm's way when being threatened with bodily injury or loss of life.

Follow-up

The captain should have notified a supervisor immediately following this event. Depending on the reactions of the crew members, it may be helpful to go out of service for a short time and debrief the call. Being threatened with a weapon is a critical incident for any EMS crew. The management and the crew members should monitor each other for signs of a stress reaction. It is also important for each crew member to document what had happened on this call.

In this case, the engine crew should follow up with the ambulance crew. They should debrief the call together and use this as a learning opportunity to increase their knowledge of the cultural beliefs and attitudes that exist on the reservation. The management of both agencies should also look at the dispatch policies. If possible, it may be helpful to send an officer from the reservation on every call when an outside agency is dispatched to the reservation.

Summary

This case demonstrates the necessity of keeping safety as the top priority. It is easy to become hyper-focused on rescue and resuscitation activities that we lose sight of the safety risks. In this case, the safety risk was very apparent. The difficulty is that the cultural issues conflicted with EMS protocols and standard operating procedures. EMS responders and their management should understand that circumstances may dictate a deviation from the protocols or the procedures.

This case also illustrates the need for agencies that respond together to be familiar with how each agency operates. In some jurisdictions, agencies that respond together have taken steps to make sure that their operating procedures are very similar or, in some cases, are the same. Taking this step reduces the chances of disagreement and conflict at an emergency scene.

EMS agencies should take measures to build the cultural competence of their employees. This can be accomplished by bringing in speakers/trainers who are members of minority groups, creating networking opportunities, not allowing stereotyping to occur, encouraging self-exploration, and focusing on team work and organizational values (Thomas, 2005).

Key Terms

Cultural Differences   This term reflects the differences among the people who EMS agencies serve. It also represents the differences found among EMS providers.

Homogenous   Being of one common derivation. Everything is the same.

Mutual Assistance/Mutual Aid Contract   A formal contract between two or more agencies that provide the same services. This agreement grants permission for any and all participants to respond into the other's jurisdiction when their services are requested.

Patient Abandonment   The discontinuation of medical treatment at a time when continuing care would normally be required.

Standard of Care   The measure of judgment and carefulness required of an EMS provider who is under a duty of care.

Scene Safety   Procedures, protocols, and practices directed at determining whether, and ensuring that, a scene is safe for emergency response intervention. These considerations range from body substance isolation (BSI) to physical threats such as criminal activity in progress, to hazardous materials spills, to power lines down, and to any other circumstance that may prove harmful to emergency services personnel working at the scene.

References

Thomas, K. (2005). *Diversity Dynamics in the Workplace*. Belmont, CA: Thomson Wadsworth.

The Perfect Storm

Psychosocial, Ethical, and Leadership Dimensions

- Community Relations
- Compassion Fatigue
- Customer Service
- Health and Wellness
- Interpersonal Skills
- Mission Focus
- Patient Advocacy
- Team Dynamics

The Perfect Storm

The sunny spring day was off to an excellent start. The rig had been washed, the quarters cleaned, and the all-important menu had been planned. The four-person paramedic engine company jumped on big red and was heading to the grocery store.

"Channel 6-EMS assignment. Difficulty breathing." The address followed and the company immediately identified it as their first due.

"Engine 4 responding," responded the captain/EMT on the rig radio. It was at this point that the clouds started to gather, and unbeknownst to them, the company was rapidly racing into the perfect storm. The chatter started almost immediately.

"I can't believe anyone could have difficulty breathing on a beautiful clear day like today. I just wish that one time we could shop for chow without somebody needing us."

"Why can't they just leave us alone?"

Upon arrival, the EMS equipment was retrieved from the compartments and the two EMTs and two paramedics made their way up the driveway. While knocking on the carport door and trying the knob, the paramedic barked, "Fire Department!" Once they were inside, it was clear why someone might be experiencing difficulty breathing. A cloud of cigarette smoke puffed out the door, and inside the smoke was visible and looked to be from ceiling to floor. The paramedic made entry first followed closely by the captain/EMT.

"Don't you know that smoking can kill you?" the paramedic asked. He followed with, "We're going to have to move you outside. It's too smoky for us to work in here."

In a gravelly voice, the elderly woman sitting at the kitchen table replied, "I'm not going outside where all the neighbors can see me!"

To this the captain replied, "It's OK Ma'am, it's beautiful and clear out. Your carport is covered and I'll even set a chair out there for you."

"I'm not going outside!" was her only reply.

"If you won't come outside, we are not going to treat you!" added the paramedic.

With a bit of firm but considerate assistance, the patient was finally moved to the carport. Her vital signs were fine, she was speaking in full sentences, and the primary and secondary medical surveys indicated that there was nothing life threatening about her condition.

"Ma'am, we can't find anything wrong with you. Do you want to go to the hospital?" the captain queried.

"Yes I want to go to the hospital. I'm not breathing right!"

"Well if you didn't smoke three packs a day, you'd probably be able to breathe," the second paramedic chimed in. The scene continued to deteriorate and the fourth member of the crew, a probationary firefighter/EMT, slowly retreated to the fire truck.

Problem Solving

What Do You Know?

- Describe what you know about this incident.

What Do You Need to Know?

- What additional information is required before further decision making?

Resources

- What potential resources would be helpful at this stage?

Responsibilities

- What legal, ethical, organizational, or interpersonal responsibilities should you consider?

Action Plan

- Decide what you would do next if you were in this situation.

Justification of Your Action Plan

- Explain the rationale you used for your decision.

Follow-up

- Would your action plan require any follow-up? Why or why not?

▓▒░▒▓ The Rest of the Story

At this point, the captain made a critical judgment. "Ma'am, we can't find anything wrong with you and I can't justify tying up an emergency transport. I can get you a general transport nonemergency ride but you'll have to wait at least 30 minutes. Or you can ask your neighbor for a ride."

"That's unacceptable," the patient retorted, raising her voice.

"Ma'am, the ambulance that is here is for those who really need it. You are not the only person in this area. What if Tommy was drowning down the street? How would you feel if you took his ambulance?"

The war of wills was now in full force. Gail force wails of discontent filled the air. A neighbor intervened and was quickly dismissed to the sidelines. The captain offered to call his boss, stubbornly sticking to his decision. The patient was finally taken away by the ambulance that had arrived on the scene and everyone involved in the altercation was very frustrated.

Subsequently, the patient called fire department headquarters to complain about how she was treated. A full investigation of the captain and crew's conduct was undertaken. After an investigation, spanning several months, including the consideration of a suspension, this case was settled. The captain and a battalion chief went to the patient's home and the captain apologized for how he and his crew treated the patient. In admitting just how poorly the incident was handled, and regretting the breakdown, the captain had this to say, "I don't mind apologizing to anyone when I am wrong. My only regret is that the department took 6 months to arrive at a simple apology. We didn't need 6 months to determine what a successful conclusion would be. We should've been able to draw this conclusion in about 6 seconds."

During the apology, the captain found out that the elderly woman's husband had died a few months before her 9-1-1 call. It became obvious that she was still grieving over her loss and really wasn't prepared to deal with the challenges that the crew's behavior elicited.

Discussion

- Where did the storm begin in this scenario?
- How did this perfect storm come about?
- What responsibility did the captain have in this scenario?
- What responsibility did the crew have during this incident?
- How does team behavior break down like this?
- What strategies can a team employ to prevent total team breakdown?
- Should a chief officer have been notified? Why or why not?
- What disciplinary action(s) should be taken, individually and/or collectively?

Skill Building

The less than desirable outcome of this call was determined at the time it was dispatched. The crew members set the tone through their expression of their collective frustration with being interrupted during grocery shopping. Attitude is everything. The time spent during response should be utilized to check everyone's attitude and focus on the mission. This attitude check is the responsibility of the captain. The company officer sets the tone, not only on the scene but en route to a scene and during preparation for response. In this case, the company officer did not serve as the solution; he became part of the problem. He hopefully knew better, yet he still chose to enter the fray.

Emergency medical service (EMS) and fire/EMS crews respond as a team. Each member has a personal responsibility to present a positive and professional attitude. Furthermore, each team member also has a responsibility to the team. When things are not going well and the interpersonal exchange becomes unprofessional, team members should intervene in the interest of the individual, the patient, and their agency.

Individual behavioral breakdowns are not excusable but are understandable. When the total team's professional behavior breaks down, it is often caused by a number of variables. The crew may have been working together too long and adopted a negative team persona. Perhaps the team was collectively burned out. Primarily, team behavior breaks down because none of the members are monitoring attitudes. When time allows, team members should check in with each other at shift change in an effort to see how everyone is doing, did they get enough rest, is everything going alright at home? If a crew member is experiencing a rough time, it is very easy to pass this along to the citizens and patients. All crew members, including probationary members, should feel empowered to intervene when attitude is concerned.

In situations that may be progressing poorly, it is always advisable to request the presence of a supervisor. Often the presence of a super visor will provide the catalyst that will turn a call around. Furthermore, the presence of a supervisor can validate the possibility that the customer is not always right or that the EMS provider is not providing adequate customer service.

Finally, disciplinary action is more than likely appropriate in this case. Discipline would best be served if the company officer was called to task. His personal actions were unacceptable and appropriate steps must be taken to prohibit any further recurrence. The company officer or crew supervisor sets the tone and must be held accountable for the crew's attitudes and actions. As the company officer sets a positive and professional tone through his or her actions, an environment of acceptable behavior is established and therefore all others present can be held accountable to that standard.

Lessons Learned

What Do You Know?

A fire/EMS crew was dispatched to a residence for a patient complaining of difficulty breathing. For a variety of possible reasons, their collective attitude was not positive. They found the patient sitting at the kitchen table near the exterior door leading to a covered carport. The patient was smoking and a considerable volume of smoke filled the room. One of the paramedics requested that the patient put her cigarette out and come out to the carport for an assessment. She refused and an ugly altercation ensued. The patient was eventually transported to the hospital. She filed a complaint about the manner in which she was treated and an investigation followed.

What Do You Need to Know?

It would be beneficial to know if this organization acknowledged the condition known as compassion fatigue and monitored personnel in an effort to address it. It would also be helpful to know if this agency has a policy requiring that the next level of supervision be called to the scene in the event of an altercation with a member of the public. Finally, was it a standard practice to require that a nonemergent patient wait for a nonemergent ambulance or did practice require that each caller be treated and transported on a first come, first served basis?

Resources

The most important, and readily available, resource that this crew had was each other. Had even one of them maintained a professional attitude and served as a patient advocate, the outcome would have probably been at least marginally positive. Rather than offering to call his supervisor, the captain should have called him. Often, a third party can mediate conflict and reach an acceptable outcome.

Responsibilities

As professional fire/EMS responders, this crew was obligated to respond, assess, treat, and possibly transport this patient. This is their mission and they have a legal and ethical responsibility to execute it. When evaluating this from an organizational perspective, some questions come to mind. Is an employee assistance program (EAP) available for employees who may need assistance in dealing with compassion fatigue and other emotional issues that impact their ability to effectively serve the public? Do the organization's policies, procedures, and practice provide for a mechanism to address customer needs in situations that are not going well? Do crew supervisors and crew members feel empowered to demand certain behaviors and actions from patients and families or is the attitude of the organization one that espouses "the customer is always right"?

All that aside, this crew did not fulfill their collective responsibility to utilize their interpersonal skills to deal effectively with conflict, build community relations, and work for successful and positive encounter outcomes.

Action Plan

The best action plan in this case would have been one of friendly compromise directed at addressing, first, the patient's immediate medical needs; second, the patient's comfort; and third, the patient's need to feel safe and cared for. It is easy to look ahead to the desired outcome and adjust the current circumstances toward the desired outcome. An action plan that remains focused on the overall mission and is directed at obtaining a win-win outcome is the practical and professional manner in which to approach even the most challenging situations.

In this scenario, the damage has already been done and the organization's attention must be directed at repairing the damage. Is punishment and disciplinary action required in this case? Maybe yes, maybe no. If the goal is to rectify the patient's complaint, then punishment and discipline are several steps down the road. It is advisable to take care of the patient's complaint. Rectify the complainant's concerns first, then move to discipline and punishment in an effort to prevent future occurrences.

Justification of Your Action Plan

Action plans should always start with a positive patient outcome as the overarching goal. When things go poorly and the outcome is in doubt, every service provider should revert to their professional responsibilities as EMS providers and patient advocates. No justification exists for an outcome such as the initial one in this scenario. However, justification does exist for an after-the-fact plan that incorporates rectifying the complaint and addressing the actions of the crew. Although the actions were reactive, rather than proactive, they led back to common ground and satisfaction on the part of the patient.

Follow-up

Patient follow-up did turn out to be a component of successfully rectifying this situation. Had follow-up, rather than an investigation, been undertaken immediately, this complaint could have been rectified within 1 or 3 days rather than 6 months. Follow-up with this supervisor and the crew would also be necessary. In this case, the follow-up included moving the supervisor to another fire station with a company officer who would hopefully provide a more positive leadership model. Additional follow-up on the part of the organization may include a more in-depth examination of compassion fatigue at the agency and individual levels.

Summary

Responding personnel must be aware that nonemergent patients come with the territory. Don't be judgmental. Many of those who call for service are doing things that we know are not good for them. People do continue to smoke, use drugs and abuse alcohol, drive recklessly, and place themselves in harm's way. It is also important that we don't attempt to define what an emergency is and what it is not. That privilege belongs to the individual calling for assistance.

It is also important to remember that not everyone shares the same values. We are often called to provide service to those who live differently than we do. During the course of a career, we are likely to provide service in homes that are smoky, unkempt, cluttered, dirty, or even infested with vermin. While we may not choose to live in these conditions, we should not judge those who do. We do not know the circumstances that have lead to these conditions.

No matter what the circumstances, emergency responders should always keep customer service and community relations as a primary focus. Community relations are an essential component of maintaining the public's trust. Positive community relations will pay great dividends when it comes to budget increases and the agency's relationship with elected officials. Community relations also determine an agency's reputation among its peers. Community relations suffer when EMS agencies do not emphasize its importance or when they do not do a good job of taking care of their employees. Agencies that allow their employees to become burned out run the risk of a deteriorating relationship with those who they serve.

Compassion fatigue must be monitored at the individual, crew, and organizational levels. A variety of programs and strategies can be implemented to prevent it. However, in all cases, those serving at the service delivery of the continuum must remain focused on the mission, serve as patient advocates, deliver sound customer services, and seek to utilize their interpersonal skills in a manner that consistently seeks and achieves desirable outcomes.

Key Terms

Community Relations   The process of building political and public support within the organization, the emergency response system, with policy makers and with the community.

Compassion Fatigue   Commonly referred to as "burnout," this term describes individuals usually working in the helping professions who have, for various reasons, lost their ability to effectively manage their personal and professional relationships with work team members, family members, supervisors, and those they serve. This is frequently caused by being overworked, continual exposure to the negative aspects of the human condition, and fatigue including sleep deprivation.

Customer Service   The process and practice of delivering services. From the fire/EMS and EMS perspective, this is usually defined as the manner in which services are delivered that produces a positive outcome.

Professionalism   Actions in the workplace that exhibit high standards of performance, dedication, and commitment to the successful completion of a given mission.

28

Family Ties

Psychosocial, Ethical, and Leadership Dimensions

- Grief
- Interagency Cooperation
- Interpersonal Skills
- Mission Focus
- Patient Advocacy

▓▓▓▓▓ **Family Ties**

The victim was obviously dead. The shotgun that he had used to destroy his head and chest had made sure of that. While it is often difficult for the living to understand suicide, for some reason this elderly man had selected suicide as his solution. Law enforcement had arrived on the scene before the dispatch of the ambulance and fire department. Upon arrival, both crews encountered two police officers blocking the door.

"No need for you guys in there," they were told by one of the officers. "He pretty much blew his head off."

Two paramedics were allowed in to run an EKG strip, so that they could confirm death with the base hospital physician. Both units went available and headed back to quarters. When the engine company had almost reached their station, they were contacted by dispatch and asked to respond back to the scene for a man down. They wondered what could be happening on the scene and were not prepared for what they encountered upon their arrival.

As the engineer/paramedic set the parking brake on the engine, they viewed a young man with his hands and legs bound behind his back in the "hog-tied" position. He was lying, squirming, and screaming in the narrow trailer park street. "He raised me! He's like my father! Let me go I've got to see him!" he yelled over and over.

"What's up?" the captain/ EMT asked the first police officer he encountered.

"Well, we're arresting this man for assaulting a police officer," he replied. "We need you guys to look at the officer's injuries."

During the assessment of the officer's very minor injuries, the situation began to unfold. Across the narrow street, a young woman, who was later identified as the perpetrator's wife, was crying and screaming, "Let him go! He didn't do anything wrong!"

Problem Solving

What Do You Know?

- Describe what you know about this incident.

What Do You Need to Know?

- What additional information is required before further decision making?

Resources

- What potential resources would be helpful at this stage?

Responsibilities

- What legal, ethical, organizational, or interpersonal responsibilities should you consider?

Action Plan

- Decide what you would do next if you were in this situation.

Justification of Your Action Plan

- Explain the rationale you used for your decision.

Follow-up

- Would your action plan require any follow-up? Why or why not?

The Rest of the Story

The captain/EMT asked further questions in an attempt to understand how and why a police officer had been assaulted at the scene of a suicide.

"It was like this," said one officer. "This guy," pointing to the man rolling and screaming in the street, "came screeching up in his car, then started charging up the walkway screaming that the dead man inside was his grandfather and that he had to see him. We told him as he was charging us that this was a crime scene and that nobody could make entry. He just kept on charging and knocked my partner to the ground. He just wouldn't let up."

"Look, why don't you just let the guy go?" asked one of the crew members. "You're not really hurt and this guy has shown us how much his grandfather meant to him."

"Sorry. This guy assaulted a police officer and he's being arrested," replied the officer.

The captain/EMT pressed his point, "The guy is out of his mind. He is consumed with grief. He's just lost one of the most important people in his life, give him a break."

"Nope, if this was one of your people, you'd want us to arrest him," the officer responded.

"No, my people are smart enough to understand the circumstances and would want to cut the guy some slack," the captain/EMT stated raising his voice.

"Well, we have a job to do and this guy is going down for assaulting a police officer," the on-scene police lieutenant stated, working his way toward those involved in the heated discussion.

Always one to have the last word, the captain/EMT angrily replied, "Well this is exactly why you are the endeared public servants that you are!"

This verbal confrontation resulted in a complaint being filed by the on-scene lieutenant. An investigation was undertaken resulting in a formal reprimand being placed in the captain's personnel file.

Discussion

- Where did the breakdowns in this situation occur?
- Is it an appropriate role for fire or emergency medical service (EMS) responders to serve as patient advocates in certain situations?
- Is this scenario one of those times?

- Did the captain/EMT handle this situation properly? Why or why not?
- How would you react to this situation?

Skill Building

The goal of interagency cooperation between law enforcement, fire, and EMS extends far beyond strict interpretation of each agency's official role. True interagency cooperation is constructed from the street up. We should make an effort to better understand the jobs and responsibilities of those we respond with, from their perspective not ours. This is fostered through dialogue and building relationships. Invite officers for dinner at your quarters. Encourage them to take their breaks and write their reports in the comfort of your station. Build a relationship with them. Ask questions and, most importantly, listen. Their perception of their role and the challenges they face are quite possibly very different than what you perceive them to be.

Had the captain been able to keep a clear head and control his emotional interpretation of the event, he may have been better able to think more rationally. He may have been able to initiate a strategy that might have led to a satisfactory outcome, rather than the negative outcome that occurred. Public servants are, as the title describes, citizen advocates. EMS responders should serve as patient advocates but must do so within professional standards and EMS protocols. It may have been possible and reasonable to make the young man in the street a patient. By doing so, the EMS responders would have established at least partial control over the grieving man's immediate destiny, perhaps calming him down and even getting the officers to release him from his restraints. Even if the young man was later charged, this approach would have provided a more positive outcome for all involved.

The young man hog-tied in the street demonstrated just how powerful grief can be. Grief can be described as an intense emotional state associated with the loss of someone or something of significance.

Every person grieves in a unique and individual way and their reaction is directly affected by their own life history (Thomas & Woodall, 2006). With this in mind, it is easy to understand the young man and his reaction. We should all make a concerted effort to understand and empathize with the challenges that those we serve are experiencing. This knowledge and understanding can be achieved through further self-study, training, and education.

The captain/EMT did not handle this situation properly. He most certainly had the right to request that the young man be untied. However, when his request was refused, he should have deferred to the officers. Engaging in a verbal confrontation did not and could not lead to a positive outcome. His actions only served to erode the working relationship with his agency and law enforcement.

Lessons Learned

What Do You Know?

A four-person ALS fire/EMS crew had been dispatched, for a second time, to the scene of an apparent suicide. This first time was to confirm a death and provide documentation of the incident. The second time was to assess the injuries received during an altercation with the dead man's grandson. The crew returned to find that the officer's injuries were minor but was quite upset that the victim's grandson was hog-tied, face down in the middle of the street.

They examined and treated the officer and also strongly, and possibly inappropriately, made some suggestions that the young man in the street be released and not charged. This led to a verbal confrontation between the company officer and the police department lieutenant. The verbal altercation led to a written complaint being filed on the fire/EMS captain.

What Do You Need to Know?

In the interest of a long-term solution, it would be helpful to know more about the interagency cooperation dynamics between the police and fire departments. Is this an isolated incident driven more by individual personalities or is it an indication of a further eroding relationship between these departments? Is this a police or EMS scene? Did the EMS responders adhere to the agency's standard operating procedures (SOPs)? This information would be critical when identifying and implementing an action plan directed at preventing this type of situation in the future.

Resources

As soon as the situation started to evolve in a bad direction, the fire/EMS captain should have sought the services of the next highest rank. The resources that would have prevented this scenario are, for the most part, intangible. While the police department may have overreacted, they were well within the law when they took the actions they did. The fire/EMS department's actions, however, exceeded their responsibilities. The fire/EMS personnel and the captain in particular should have called on their mission focus, SOPs, and EMS protocols to assist them in their decision making.

If the fire/EMS department utilizes the services of a chaplain, victim assistance, or other counseling/social services–type agencies, that service could be very helpful to assist the surviving family members. They could have also possibly served as an advocate for the young man in the street.

Responsibilities

Law enforcement and fire/EMS have the responsibility to cooperate smoothly and effectively in the interest of mitigating emergencies, all the while working within the incident command system (ICS). It is true that their responsibilities often overlap creating the potential for conflict. The on-scene individuals also have the responsibility to the organization they represent and must comply with protocols, policies, and procedures. In this case, the young man hog-tied in the street had not been identified as a patient. Therefore, his welfare was not the responsibility of the fire/EMS crew. Interpersonally, all emergency responders have the responsibility to employ their interpersonal skills in a professional manner while in the workplace and on the emergency scene.

Action Plan

Although the position of the captain and his crew could be considered noble, it did not reflect a strong mission focus. An action plan that would have avoided this outcome would include answering some very basic questions on the part of the captain and crew: What is the specific mission on this call? Who is our patient? And, what are my responsibilities in regard to EMS protocols, SOPs, and the law? Answering these questions would lead them to some very basic answers: My patient is the officer whom we've been asked to assess. My job is to treat the officer following our assigned EMS protocols and SOPs. The police department enforces the law.

Justification of Your Action Plan

Whether right or wrong, the fire/EMS captain and his crew should have avoided this conflict. A plan grounded in the basics, interagency cooperation, mission focus, and following protocols, policies, and procedures is the only justifiable plan.

Follow-up

Follow-up in this case would include a case review with the fire/EMS crew discussing where this had gone wrong, why it had gone so poorly, and how it could be avoided in the future. A comprehensive prevention plan would also include a discussion with the police department with the hopes of repairing interagency cooperation.

Summary

These responders were witnessing a severe grief reaction. The young man in the street was delirious and out of control. It was difficult for these compassionate public servants to control their desire to assist him. They assumed the role of patient advocate even though he was not their patient.

Compassion, understanding, and empathy are important qualities in EMS responders. The ability to employ these interpersonal skills is what makes this human services profession human. We shouldn't lose these qualities and we certainly don't want to ignore them. However, these qualities must certainly be measured, managed, and controlled, as they can often cloud our judgment resulting in actions that can trip us up and make us fall. We would all be wise to guard against allowing our personal belief systems to lead us down an emotionally charged path.

Finally, the missions of fire/EMS and law enforcement do frequently overlap. It is important to understand this and be very careful about not crossing these often ambiguous boundaries. In the post–September 11 world, our ability to work effectively with other agencies is more important than it has ever been. We, the agencies charged with the safety and welfare of our citizens, must constantly seek to build relationships that lead to and foster interagency cooperation.

Key Terms

Grief   An intense emotional state associated with the loss of someone (or something) with whom (or which) one has had a deep emotional bond (Reber, 1995).

Interagency Cooperation   The collaboration of more than one agency to meet a specified objective.

Interpersonal skills   Those skills and abilities that allow a person to successfully interact with others.

References

Reber, A. S. (1995). *The Penguin Dictionary of Psychology*, 2nd ed. New York, NY: Penguin Books Ltd.

Thomas, J., & Woodall, S. J. (2006). *Responding to Psychological Emergencies: A Field Guide*. Clifton Park, NY: Delmar-Thomson Learning.

Salute

Psychosocial, Ethical, and Leadership Dimensions

- Death
- Diversity
- Grief

░░░░░ **Salute**

The crew of Engine 30 was busy washing their truck one morning when they were dispatched to an EMS call for an unconscious person. The mobile computer terminal indicated that a 47-year-old man had not gotten out of bed this morning and that his family members had been unable to awaken him. The address was not far away and they took some small comfort knowing that they would be there in just a couple of minutes.

When they arrived, there was a small crowd of people at the front door. The firefighters grabbed their equipment while the captain radioed dispatch and asked them to send a police unit to the scene. The people at the front door were all talking and yelling frantically. Some of them were speaking English and some were speaking in a language that the captain did not recognize.

A family member ushered the crew past another group of people gathered in the living room and into a front bedroom. There they found a Caucasian male lying supine under the bedcovers. His skin was pale and cold to the touch. There was no pulse and he was not breathing. The paramedics quickly hooked up the monitor and determined that there was indeed no heartbeat. They rolled the patient on his side. His limbs were beginning to stiffen and there were signs of lividity. By this time, two police officers had arrived on the scene. The paramedics contacted the base hospital and were given permission to pronounce the man dead. They explained to the family that there was nothing to be done and expressed their condolences.

This news spread quickly to the family members in the living room and to those standing outside the front door. The women began wailing and sobbing. The men began to talk urgently among themselves in the unrecognizable language. As the fire crew gathered the equipment, the police officers secured the bedroom for the coroner. Soon they were all standing in the living room with the family. Before they knew what was happening, the firefighters and the police officers were each handed a shot glass as a male member of the family walked around and filled each glass from a bottle of clear liquor.

When the man got to the captain, the captain politely declined explaining that the firefighters and the police officers were all on duty and were not allowed to consume alcohol. The man insisted and the captain was forced to refuse a second time. By now the room had grown silent and the entire family was staring at the firefighters and police officers with disbelief. One of the older women said something in the foreign language while making a face of disgust. Finally, another man explained in broken English that it was customary in his country for everyone to have a drink and salute the deceased family member, everyone including the police officers and the firefighters.

Problem Solving

What Do You Know?
- Describe what you know about this incident.

What Do You Need to Know?
- What additional information would be helpful before further decision making?

Resources
- What potential resources would be helpful at this stage?

Responsibilities
- What legal, ethical, organizational, or interpersonal responsibilities should you consider?

Action Plan
- Decide what you would do next if you were in this situation.

Justify Your Action Plan
- Explain the rationale you used for your decision.

Follow-up

- Would your action require any follow-up? Why or why not?

🔲 The Rest of the Story

After an awkward silence, the captain suggested that they participate by raising their empty shot glasses. Although the family seemed disappointed with this solution, they agreed and everyone raised their glass in salute. The Engine 30 crew again expressed their condolences and returned to the station. All of them felt a bit uneasy about what had just transpired with that family.

Discussion

- Did the Engine 30 crew violate standard emergency medical service (EMS) protocols?
- Why do you think the family was initially offended?
- Are you aware of any different customs regarding death that are prevalent in your community?
- Suggest some other strategies that these paramedics could have used in this situation.

Skill Building

The Engine 30 crew members did not violate any standard EMS protocols. It was clearly evident that the patient was deceased and they contacted their base hospital before pronouncing him dead. After receiving the news, the family began to participate in a death ritual that was customary in their culture. Many times our customers are from different countries where the cultural norms are very different from our own. It is entirely possible that both police officers and firefighters in another country would have consumed the alcohol without giving it a second thought. If the family members were unaware of the rules and regulations that prohibit emergency service personnel in the United

States from consuming alcohol on duty, they could have interpreted the captain's refusal as a sign of disrespect. It is important to respect other cultures by acknowledging and participating in its death rituals in whatever way we can. Perhaps the officers and the firefighters could have filled their glasses with water or Gatorade and symbolically drank that in a salute to the deceased. If the crew was not entirely comfortable with the outcome of this encounter, they could have followed-up with the family the next shift or asked to have the chaplain or some other member of their agency to call on the family and express condolences.

It is also important to remember that EMS professionals, firefighters, and police officers are perceived differently by people of different cultures. Some people may not be accustomed to granting the high level of respect that emergency responders are granted in our society. In some instances, they may be very suspicious and mistrusting of emergency responders or any government official. There are countries where people in uniform are considered dangerous and are feared by the public. These beliefs can lead to awkward moments when providing emergency medical care. Responders can counteract some of this by being sensitive to cultural issues, keeping an open mind, and taking the opportunity to educate those members of our society who may have grown up with different belief systems.

Lessons Learned

What Do You Know?

Engine 30 responded to a private residence close to their station for an unconscious party. They were informed en route that a 47-year-old man had not gotten out of bed and his family was unable to awaken him. When they arrived on scene, a crowd of people were gathered at the front door. The captain requested a police unit. The living room was also full of people. Most of them were speaking a foreign language that the crew did not recognize.

The paramedics examined the patient who had clearly been dead for some time. They contacted the base hospital and were given permission to pronounce him dead at the scene. After informing the family that the man had died, the family began grieving and a bustle of activity started. Each of the firefighters and the police officers were handed a shot glass and expected to drink a toast to the man who died. When the captain politely refused, the people in the home were offended. Eventually, the police officers and the firefighters participated in the toast by raising their empty glasses.

What Do You Need to Know?

Many cultures have death rituals that are different from the majority culture. These differences include beliefs regarding the meaning of death and a hereafter, funeral rites, and methods of caring for the dead. In some societies, there is a strong social significance directed to the dead, the dying, and the bereaved. It is important to respect these differences.

Resources

Since the captain saw that there was a crowd of people at the front door of the house, he was wise to call for police assistance. Crowd behavior can be unpredictable and it is better to have a resource there that is not needed rather than need one and have it not be there. If the department has a chaplain, this may have been a good time to request a response. In this case, the police department may also have had a chaplain. Some jurisdictions also have specialized units that can give assistance to grieving family members.

Responsibilities

Since the patient was clearly deceased, nothing could be done. If the police department had not been on scene, they would have to be notified. The bedroom should be secured so that the coroner can conduct an investigation. We also have the responsibility to care for and give emotional first aid to the family and friends of the deceased.

Action Plan

The responders in this case did everything they could. They secured the bedroom for the coroner. They did not consume the alcohol but did find a way to participate in the ritual.

Justify Your Action Plan

Emergency responders are not allowed to consume alcohol while on duty. This would be a violation of their agency's policies and would likely result in disciplinary action.

Follow-up

If the crew was still feeling uncomfortable, they could visit the family during their next shift. They could also send the family something like a plate of cookies. Most cultures recognize the giving of food as a gesture of caring and compassion.

Summary

The crew in this case did everything right. Despite this fact, they still felt uncomfortable. Emergency responders often find themselves in uncomfortable or awkward situations. It may be useful to view these situations as opportunities for professional development. Through this experience, the crew learned something about how people from another culture handle the death of a family member.

Responding to a call where there is loss of life can be one of the most difficult parts of EMS providers' job. Treating patients who do not survive is contrary to the basic premise of EMS. We should not view these instances as negative outcomes. Death is a part of the life cycle. It is also important to remember that even in the face of death we still have the opportunity to help the living. Providing comfort and emotional first aid is a significant and valuable service.

Sometimes being around death can remind us of our losses and trigger a grief reaction. This is a normal human reaction. Talking about grief and loss is essential to emotional health. Emergency responders should talk about these feelings with someone they trust. This could be a coworker, a family member, or a friend. Other resources include employee assistance programs (EAP), mental health professionals, and members of the clergy. By not addressing these feelings when they come up, we run the risk of developing compassion fatigue, becoming burned out, or developing a stress-related disorder.

Key Terms

Belief Systems   A framework of ideas, philosophies, and values that an individual uses to interpret the world and his or her behavior as well as the behavior of others.

Compassion Fatigue   Commonly referred to as "burnout," this term describes individuals usually working in the helping professions who have, for various reasons, lost their ability to effectively manage their personal and professional relationships with work team members, family members, supervisors, and those they serve. This is frequently caused by being overworked, continual exposure to the negative aspects of the human condition, and fatigue including sleep deprivation.

Condolences   An expression of sympathy.

Employee Assistance Program   A benefit program provided by the employer who usually offers assessment, short-term counseling, and referral services.

Funeral Rites   A ceremony marking a person's death.

In Their Time of Grief

Psychosocial, Ethical, and Leadership Dimensions

- Community Relations
- Customer Service
- Grief
- Standard Operating Procedures

In Their Time of Grief

The crew was hot, tired, and hungry after returning from a fire just before sundown on a hot summer night. They knew they had done an outstanding job, and as a fire department truck company, they took great pride in their performance. As they headed for the firehouse in anticipation of another savory meal that their housemate engine company was preparing, they discussed the fire, their performance, what went well, and what could have gone better. They were also trying to remember what was on the menu and, most importantly, who was doing the cooking. They all hoped that the best firehouse cook, "Jimmy the Fish," was at the kitchen controls.

Suddenly, off to their left, a dog broke free from its leash and darted onto the busy street. Before anyone could say a word, the dog was struck by a car. They witnessed, firsthand, the panic on the faces of the mom, dad, and their two children—a boy about 10 and his sister about 8. Just seconds before, this family had been peacefully and happily walking the family pet, probably going to the corner store for some ice cream.

The crew instinctively and immediately pulled over. They checked the traffic and jumped off to retrieve the flailing but dying dog. They also took actions to protect the distraught family whose members were in peril from the traffic as they tried to help their mortally wounded family member. When, at last, they were able to intervene, it was obvious that the dog's injuries were fatal and their mission had shifted from the usual one of providing care to that of offering condolences and support.

The family members, especially the young kids, were beside themselves—crying, screaming, and wailing as they came to realize their loved one was gone forever. Without gesture, without spoken words, without a second thought, they all moved into action. The two firefighter/EMTs on the crew gently removed the dog from the street, placing it carefully and respectfully on the sidewalk. The engineer and the captain went to the family, consoling them and offering their assistance. As they brought a semblance of organization to the hectic and tragic scene, it became apparent that their job was not done. They simply could not leave this family alone on the street.

Problem Solving

What Do You Know?

- Describe what you know about this incident.

What Do You Need to Know?

- What additional information would be helpful before further decision making?

Resources

- What potential resources would be helpful at this stage?

Responsibilities

- What legal, ethical, organizational, or interpersonal responsibilities should you consider?

Action Plan

- Decide what you would do next if you were in this situation.

Justification of Your Action Plan

- Explain the rationale you used for your decision.

Follow-up

- Would your action plan require any follow-up? Why or why not?

The Rest of the Story

The captain asked the family where they lived and volunteered to take the whole family home. Upon their acceptance, the crew placed the dog on the extended front bumper of the truck and helped the mom, dad, and kids into the truck. All the seats were taken, so a crew member and the captain sat on the front bumper with the deceased canine. They slowly drove the one-truck funeral procession toward the family's home, less than a block into the residential area. Upon reaching the family's home, condolences, hugs, and thanks were exchanged. The family was extremely grateful, and the father told them how much he appreciated their efforts to make a tragic situation a little bit better.

The gratification they received by helping this family in their time of extreme need far outweighed the satisfaction they had received from their most recent fire-ground performance. The captain of this great crew had enjoyed many moments in which he had beamed with pride over their performance, but none provided him with deeper satisfaction and pride than the compassionate and thoughtful way in which these men instinctively reacted to an extremely unfortunate situation.

Discussion

- Were any standard operating procedures (SOPs) violated?
- If so, was the captain justified in choosing to breach a SOP? Why or why not?
- Should a supervisor have been notified? Why or why not?
- Does this represent exemplary customer service?

Skill Building

We provide our emergency responders with the latest tools, equipment, and training. These efforts are directed toward sending them into the field to solve a wide and growing variety of challenges. As organizations, we attempt to regulate these responses with SOPs and protocols. In most cases, these policies and the approach to service delivery derived from them serve us well. However, we should also be aware that we cannot plan for every contingency and should keep this in mind when we attempt to script the actions of field personnel. This case exemplifies just how SOPs can sometimes prove counterproductive for field responders. Most agencies possess SOPs regulating citizen observers riding on department apparatus. These SOPs often require a preapproval form signed by an administrator. Riding outside the cab is forbidden in most, if not all, agencies. Had the SOPs been established as standard operating guidelines (SOGs), the company officer could have addressed this incident with little fear of disciplinary action.

Administrators should be cognizant that although SOPs are designed to create consistency in our technical approach to problem solving and to enhance safety, they can often serve as barriers to good customer service. A certain degree of flexibility should be built into the system to allow for creative solutions. The captain did violate a SOP but hopefully put his decision under close personal scrutiny. The captain decided to take the family home because they lived so close to the scene. Furthermore, the street on which the dog had been struck was extremely busy and therefore dangerous to the children. From an emotional well-being perspective, it was also a good idea to get the family away from the scene. And finally, home is where a family is drawn during a time of grief (Thomas & Woodall, 2006). It may have been prudent for the captain to call his supervisor. In this case, he chose not to. When possible, it is always a good idea to consult with a supervisor when a breach of SOPs is under consideration.

Actions like those taken by this crew represent the best of emergency services personnel can offer the public in their time of need. Yes, this example of exemplary customer service could have been a public relations windfall for the department but public relations had nothing to do with the actions of this crew (Brunacini, 1996). This was about empathy and sympathy. There are few among us who have not lost a pet. It is something we all understand at a deep emotional level. This crew immediately went to those emotional experiences understanding the pain and suffering the family was going through. They simply tried to make it better.

Many times organizations look to the wrong metrics when attempting to measure individual and team performance. This story epitomizes the founding principles of emergency care service delivery: a group of fellow citizens' ready, willing, and available to assist members of their community in their time of need. Those on the job understand that calls like this are the ones that are never forgotten. Those new to the profession will eventually understand that multi-alarm fires and multicar pileups are what we train for and what we like to do, but the ability to look a fellow citizen in the eyes, see their gratitude, and feel their love is what makes this job the special job that it is.

Lessons Learned

What Do You Know?

While returning from a call, this Basic Life Support (BLS) ladder company witnessed a dog being struck by a car while the family of four stood helplessly on the sidewalk. They stopped, retrieved the dying pet, and comforted the family. After the dog was obviously dead, they wrapped the dog in a plastic salvage cover, loaded the dog on the front bumper of the truck with two firefighters, placed the family in the cab of the truck, and took the family to their home.

What Do You Need to Know?

The information in this scenario is complete. We may not even know exactly why the company officer chose to stretch SOPs, but we can certainly speculate. Basically, he wanted to help a family in distress. He weighed his options and made a decision. Knowledge of the agency's ride along SOPs would be helpful in the final analysis.

Resources

If an animal control agency had been available as a resource, it would have been better equipped to handle the disposition of the dog. The shift supervisor may also have had a vehicle that could accommodate the family and the dog in a fashion that would not have violated the fire department's SOPs.

The captain may have considered asking the father and mother if there was any support resource such as a family member, pastor, preacher, rabbi, or other type of spiritual advisor who could be called. If not, and the resources were available, he may have wanted to call the agency's chaplain.

Responsibilities

There were no legal or ethical considerations in this scenario. Organizationally, this crew demonstrated that their organization cared and was sensitive to the need to help others in their time of significant need. The crew also fulfilled their interpersonal responsibilities through their actions and attitude. Even though a bit unorthodox, they acted in a manner that produced a positive outcome and represented their department in a professional manner.

Action Plan

The action plan would have conformed to SOP if they had called for alternative resources, such as an animal control agency, and consulted with their supervisor. The action plan they selected also met the immediate needs of the family and fortunately no one was harmed.

Justification of Your Action Plan

While not attempting to encourage anyone to depart from SOPs, in particular SOPs directed at the safety and welfare of personnel, it is important to emphasize that the intentions of this crew were admirable. An action plan designed to incorporate these same admirable intentions should have been determined and acted upon. Safety must be considered in every decision that is made and implemented. Taking risks, no matter how minor, are not part of a sound decision-making process.

Follow-up

Follow-up in this case would primarily focus on how this type of conflict could be avoided in the future. It is imperative that we all develop the skills and abilities to work together in settings that do not involve mass casualties, such as large-scale disasters and acts of terrorism. We must develop these practices so that in the event the big one does come our way we will have the foundational skills to effectively mitigate them. We must commit ourselves to successfully manage the small ones so that we are prepared for the big one.

Summary

This case study includes several dimensions that should be addressed. Most certainly, there is the acknowledgement that emergency responders often encounter significant others in the initial stages of grief reaction. The other factors include mitigating a situation that may be beyond the boundaries of SOPs and how we manage chaos in an effort to build positive community relations all the while following SOPs and fulfilling our common mission.

When calls for service overlap those boundaries, we must possess the ability to maintain our professionalism, focus on our particular mission, seek ways to meet the intent of the SOPs, and seek a solution that meets the needs of those we serve.

Key Terms

Grief   An intense emotional state associated with the loss of someone (or something) with whom (or which) one has had a deep emotional bond (Reber, 1995).

References

Brunacini, A. (1996). *Essentials of Fire Department Customer Service.* Stillwater, OK: Fire Protection Publication.

Reber, A. S. (1995). *The Penguin Dictionary of Psychology*, 2nd ed. New York, NY: Penguin Books Ltd.

Thomas, J., & Woodall, S. J. (2006). *Responding to Psychological Emergencies: A Field Guide.* Clifton Park, NY: Delmar-Thomson Learning.

A

Active Listening   Listening for and identifying the emotional tone of what a patient is saying. Active listening includes reflecting the feeling back to the patient. If you are incorrect, the patient will correct you. Examples include: "You sound angry," "You're frightened," "I hear the sadness in your voice." Never tell patients they shouldn't feel the way that they do.

Acute Stress Reaction   Symptoms that develop within 1 month after exposure to an extreme traumatic stressor or event. These symptoms interfere with a person's daily functioning and are not the result of other psychological disorders.

Antidepressants   A class of psychotropic medications, or other substance such as an herb or nutritional supplement, used for alleviating the symptoms of depression.

Anxiety   A vague, unpleasant emotional state with the qualities of apprehension, dread, distress, and uneasiness.

Attending   Behaviors that let patients know that you are paying attention to them. Examples of positive attending behaviors include maintaining good eye contact, using the patient's name, refraining from charting or taking notes, and giving the patient your full attention.

Attention Deficit Hyperactivity Disorder (ADD/ADHD)   A neurological condition characterized by distractibility, forgetfulness, hyperactivity, and impulse control.

Autoerotic Asphyxiation Syndrome (AEA)   Accidental death that occurs when an individual deliberately restricts the flow of oxygen to the brain while masturbating.

B

Belief Systems   A framework of ideas, philosophies, and values that an individual uses to interpret the world, their own behavior, and the behavior of other people.

Biases   A personal and sometimes unreasoned prejudice in a general or specific sense, usually in the sense for having a preference to one particular person, place, thing, or idea.

Blood Sugar Levels   The amount of glucose (sugar) in the blood; also known as serum glucose level. Normally, blood glucose levels stay within narrow limits throughout the day, but they are higher after meals and usually lowest in the morning. In diabetes the blood sugar level moves outside these limits until treated.

Brief Psychosocial History   A systematic gathering of an individual's current level of mental and social functioning.

BSI   An acronym commonly used for "Body-Substance-Isolation" that describes the actions taken by the EMS provider to ensure that those working with a patient are not unnecessarily exposed to the body substances emanating from a patient.

C

Chain of Command   The line of authority and responsibility along which orders and directives are passed within an emergency response agency.

Coin Rubbing   A legitimate treatment practice in traditional Chinese medicine

that is practiced just as much by highly trained experts as it is practiced by the folk users. It should be viewed as an immediate form of domestic first aid intervention that serves to prevent any need for further medical treatment.

Condolences   An expression of sympathy.

Confidentiality   Federal law requires that all patient information and patient records be kept confidential.

Content Paraphrase   Remarks given to a patient that let him/her know that you understand what he or she has been saying. Some suggested techniques include summarizing what the patient has told you and using quotes if appropriate.

Community Relations   The process for building political and public support within the organization, the emergency response system, with policy makers, and with the community.

Compassion Fatigue   Commonly referred to as *burn-out*, this term describes individuals usually working in the helping professions who have, for a variety of reasons, lost their ability to effectively manage their personal and professional relationships with team members, family members, supervisors, and those they serve. This is frequently caused by being over worked, continual exposure to the negative aspects of the human condition, and fatigue including sleep deprivation.

CNS Stimulants   Psychotropic medications that speed up physical and mental processes.

Critical Incident Stress Management   An adaptive short-term helping process that focuses solely on an immediate and identifiable problem to enable the individual(s) affected to return to their daily routine(s) more quickly and with a lessened likelihood of experiencing post-traumatic stress disorder.

Cultural Differences   Reflects the differences among the people that EMS agencies serve. It also represents the differences found among emergency responders.

Customer Service   The process and practice of delivering services. From the fire/EMS and EMS perspective this is usually defined as the manner in which services are delivered that produces a positive outcome.

D

D-50   Dextrose 50%. Class: Carbohydrate, hypertonic solution. The term *dextrose* is used to describe the six-carbon sugar d-glucose, the principal form of carbohydrate used by the body. D50 is used in emergency care to treat hypoglycemia and to manage coma of unknown origin.

Decompensate   A deterioration of mental state that usually leads to an increase of the signs and symptoms associated with one's condition.

Defusing   The term given to the process of talking something through.

Delusion   A belief that is maintained in spite of argument, data, and refutation that should (reasonably) be sufficient to destroy it.

Depersonalization   The sense of loss of self or of personal identity; sometimes referred to as the feeling of being on autopilot.

Detachment   The lack of feeling or emotional involvement in a problem, situation, or interactions with another person.

Developmental Disabilities   Physical or mental conditions that slow what is considered to be the normal psychological developmental process.

Despair   An emotional state characterized by the loss of all hope or confidence.

Door Openers   Comments that encourage the patient to share more information. Examples include "Tell me more," "Help me understand that," and "Explain that to me."

Discretion The quality of being discreet, especially with regard to speech or behavior.

DUI Driving under the influence of drugs or alcohol. The legal blood/alcohol limits are defined on a state-by-state basis.

DWI Driving while intoxicated on drugs or alcohol. The legal blood/alcohol limits are defined on a state-by-state basis.

E

Emotional First Aid A type of psychological intervention focused on helping people to feel calm, safe, and that they are being well cared for during an acute, critical situation.

Employee Assistance Program A benefit program provided by the employer that usually offers assessment, short-term counseling, and referral services.

EMS Protocols Guidelines for prehospital patient care.

Empathetic A cognitive awareness and understanding of the emotions and feelings of another person.

Enabling Behavior Behaviors and actions that allow others to continue dysfunctional, unethical, illegal, or harmful behavior(s).

Encounter Form The patient charting form utilized to document patient contact, medical findings, medicines, chief complaint, and other important information utilized by the receiving hospital in an effort to understand the situation and expeditiously treat a patient. This form is also used to document a coherent patient's right to refuse treatment and transportation to a medical facility. Although the content requirements of this document can vary from agency to agency, it is a legal document.

Equal Employment Opportunity Commission (EEOC) The federal agency responsible for ending employment discrimination in the United States.

ETA An acronym commonly used for 'Estimated Time of Arrival."

Ethics The ability to make sound decisions based on what is considered right and wrong, what is morale, and what is legal.

EtOH The chemical formula for ethel alcohol that is found in alcoholic beverages. This designation is frequently used in the emergency medical and law enforcement field setting to describe and document a person under the influence of alcohol.

Evidence Preservation A system of law enforcement protocols directed at preserving crime scene evidence when working at or on an active crime scene.

Exaggerated Startle Response A complex reaction to a sudden, unanticipated stimulus. The stimulus may be real or imaginary. There is flexion of most skeletal muscles and a variety of visceral and hormonal reactions.

F

Fitness for Duty The physical and mental health status of an employee that allows for the performance of essential job duties in an effective and safe manner and protects the health and safety of oneself, coworkers, and the public.

Funeral Rites A ceremony marking a person's death.

G

Grief An intense emotional state associated with the loss of someone (or something) with whom (or which) one has had a deep emotional bond.

H

Hallucination A perceptual experience with all the compelling subjective properties of a real sensory impression but without the normal physical stimulus for that sensory modality.

Healthcare System The organization and the method by which health care is provided.

HIPAA Health Insurance Portability and Accountability Act established regulations for the use and disclosure of protected health information.

Holiday Mode Fire and EMS agencies develop individual cultures. On Sundays and holidays, the crews are allowed to relax more, plan their own days, and generally recover from the rigorous Monday through Saturday schedule.

Homelessness Intentionally or unintentionally being without a permanent home that would provide for what is considered normal amenities such as a bed, a shower, a kitchen, and restroom.

Homogenous Being of one common derivation. Everything is the same.

Hostile Work Environment A hostile work environment exits when there is an offensive, intimidating, or oppressive environment.

Hypervigilance   State of being associated with extreme carefulness, awareness to the possibility of danger or injury.

I

Immediate Patient   A patient who requires rapid assessment and medical intervention for survival.

Incident Command System   A structured incident management system that is commonly employed at incidents in which span-of-control is an issue. The presence of an incident commander allows those treating the patients to focus on the task level while the incident commander directs attention to strategy, safety, and resource management issues such as hospital and patient transportation availability.

Inter-Agency Cooperation   The collaboration of more than one agency to meet a specified objective.

Interpersonal Skills   Those skills and abilities that allow a person to successfully interact with others.

L

Lethality Assessment   A systematic set of questions conducted in an effort to assess a person's determination to commit harm to himself/herself or to others.

Light Duty   Reassignment of an employee to another position, compatible with medically imposed restrictions and/or limitations.

M

Managed Care   A model in U.S. health care delivery that is intended to reduce unnecessary health care costs.

Mechanism of Injury   The process of examining evidence available on the scene in an effort to better determine and assign a triage level to a patient impacted by the mechanism. This is not an exact science but it is often utilized in cases involving patients in motor vehicle accidents. The mechanism of injury often leads to the upgrading of the medical level assigned to a patient in cases where the damage to the mechanism is severe.

Medical Alarm   An automated electronic notification device worn on, or kept near to, the subscriber. When activated, a signal is transmitted to a monitoring agency who in turn notifies the appropriate emergency medical provider.

Medical Control Decisions regarding patient treatment and transport are the responsibility of the highest-level EMS professional (paramedic, EMT, etc.) providing care to a specific patient. Medical control functions independently of the EMS professional's rank in the chain of command.

Mental Status Exam A full clinical work-up of a psychiatric patient including assessment of overall psychiatric condition, diagnosis of existing disorders, prognosis, estimates of suitability for treatment of various kinds, formulation of overall personality, compilation of historical and developmental data, etc.

Morale The capacity of people to maintain belief in an institution, a goal, or even in oneself and others.

Morbid Obesity The state of being overweight to the point that a persons normal life expectancy is greatly reduced.

Mutual Assistance/Mutual Aid Contract A formal contract between two or more agencies that provide the same services. This agreement grants permission for any and all participants to respond to the other's jurisdiction when their services are requested.

N

Noncommittal Acknowledgments Actions that let patients know you are listening to them. Examples include: nodding your head while the person is talking, vocalizations such as "ah," "uh-huh," or "hmmm," and responding with comments such as "yes," "I'm listening," or "okay."

Non-Emergent Patients Individuals who have accessed the EMS or medical system and who require medical attention but whose illness or injury is not life-threatening.

O

Open-Ended Questions Useful for gathering information regarding the emergency. A good method to use when asking an open-ended question is to ask questions that require more than a simple yes or no answer: "Tell me what has happened to you today." This method encourages patients to talk freely.

P

Parental Consent Laws that require that one or more parents' permission notification before their minor child can legally engage in certain activities such as seeking healthcare.

Pathway Management A process created by healthcare agencies that are outside of the EMS system. This system allows patients to have access to a trained healthcare professional who can assess their condition and make recommendations.

Patient Abandonment The discontinuation of medical treatment at a time when continuing care would normally be required.

Patient Advocacy The act of assuming the role of a patient representative in circumstances in which the patient is unwilling or unable to serve in his/her own best interest regarding treatment, transportation, and medical care.

Patient Modesty Respecting the needs of patients who need to be undressed for examination or need to disclose sensitive information.

Patient Refusal Form A legal document utilized in the emergency medical field setting. By understanding and signing this document the individual releases the responding individuals and their agency from any liability that may arise from the termination of their treatment and transportation to the emergency department.

Personal Safety An individual's responsibility to practice procedurally driven safety precautions that are directed at enhancing the safety of each member.

Pica A rare condition in which patients compulsively eat things not normally consumed as food.

Pilfering To steal small amounts or trivial objects.

Personal Responsibility The set of personal standards that an individual holds himself/herself to. Personal responsibility is driven by the person's belief system, world view, work ethic, and morals.

PPE An acronym commonly used for "Personal Protective Equipment." For EMS calls this equipment is comprised of latex gloves, eye protection, substance resistance pull on sleeves, gowns, and filtering masks. In fire situations, PPE would consist of turnout gear, helmet, boots, and a self-contained breathing apparatus (SCBA).

Post-Traumatic Stress Disorder (PTSD) A type of anxiety disorder that emerges after a psychologically distressing, traumatic event such as disaster, accident, war, rape, etc.

Professionalism Actions in the workplace that exhibit high standards of performance, dedication, and commitment to the successful completion of a given mission.

Professional Accountability Being responsible and answerable for the performance of one's professional duties.

Professional Courtesy An informal process in which law enforcement extends greater latitude to a fellow officer, EMS personnel, firefighters, and other public officials.

Professional Ethics Ethical positions in the workplace. A person's professional ethics are influenced by personal philosophies, beliefs, morals, and those they work with and for.

Providing Resources The conscious and specific actions taken to by an individual or an advocate to call for and secure the resources that are necessary to successfully mitigate a situation.

Psychosis Referring to the total mental condition of a person who has suffered a break from reality at a specific moment.

Psychosocial History A systematic gathering of an individual's psychological history, emotional and behavioral history, family and social supports, and current level of mental and social functioning.

Psychotic Condition Referring to the total mental condition of a person who has suffered a break from reality at a specific moment.

Psychotic Disorder Often used to describe a set of symptoms characterized by delusional thinking and/or hallucinations.

Public Education Comprehensive wellness and injury prevention programs designed to eliminate or mitigate situations that risk the lives or health of the public.

Public–Private Partnership Formal or informal interagency agreements designed to enhance a given system of service or a process in the interest of the end consumer.

Public Trust The foundation of those who govern and those who serve in the public's interest. This trust is earned through honesty, integrity, hard work, professionalism, and the delivery of competent service.

R

Refusal Form   A "refusal of treatment and transportation" form must be signed by any patient not requesting transport by ambulance. If the patient is not capable of signing the refusal because of injury to his/her writing hand/arm, etc., then the refusal must be witnessed. If the patient is not capable of signing the refusal because of an altered level of consciousness, you should reconsider whether he/she is mentally competent to refuse care.

Reporting Child Abuse   Child abuse and neglect is the subject of mandatory reporting for emergency responders in all jurisdictions.

Ride-Along   Structured programs in which citizens visit fire stations and ambulance quarters to get a better understanding of how fire departments and EMS agencies work and what fire and EMS professionals do on a daily basis. This is a process many folks use to determine if they would like to work in our field and to also learn about the job in preparation for employment tests and job interviews.

S

Scene Safety   Procedures, protocols, and practices directed at determining if, and ensuring that, a scene is safe for emergency response intervention. These considerations range from BSI to physical threats such as criminal activity in progress, to hazardous materials spills, to power lines down and any other circumstance that may prove harmful to emergency services personnel working at the scene.

Scene Size-Up   The process of assessing the emergency scene for potential hazards to ensure the safety of all patients and emergency responders at the scene, and assessing the nature and type of emergency.

Self-Disclosure   Disclosing to the patient what is happening for you at that very moment. Examples include: "I'm confused," "I don't understand," "I'm concerned about you," "I want to help you." It is inappropriate and unprofessional to share personal stories from your own life.

Sexual Harassment   Unwelcome attention or behavior of a sexual nature.

Silence Allowing time for silence gives patients time to collect their thoughts. It is not necessary to feel as though you must fill up the silence. However, if the silence is prolonged, try an open-ended question.

Sleep Deprivation Being deprived of adequate quality sleep or an extended period of time. The negative impacts of sleep deprivation are cumulative in nature and can lead to long-term health problems as well as increasing the probability of accidents and injuries.

Social Services Agencies concerned with the causes, solutions, and human impacts of social problems.

Spanglish A blend of the English-language words for Spanish and English; describes a dialect in which the speaker intermittently changes from Spanish to English and vice versa.

Standard of Care The measure of judgment and carefulness required of an EMS provider who is under a duty of care.

Standard Operating Procedure A written set of procedures that define particular tasks to be performed in a step-by-step format.

Stress Reaction Emotional and physical reactions that are manifested due to experiencing or being exposed to a disturbing and or harmful event.

Subintentional Death Behavior that indirectly and/or unconsciously causes death.

Sudden Infant Death Syndrome (SIDS) A syndrome marked by the symptoms of sudden and unexplained death of an apparently healthy infant aged 1 month to 1 year. The term *cot death* is often used in the United Kingdom, Australia, and New Zealand, while *crib death* is used in North America.

Supervision The action carried out to oversee the productivity and progress of employees who report directly to an individual.

T

Transport Protocols Every EMS system is required to develop and implement procedures governing the assessment and transportation of patients.

Triage The medical protocol driven process in which multiple patients are assessed as to the seriousness and level of treatment required. Those with life-threatening injuries are the first to be treated and transported. Those with serious injuries that are not life threatening are treated and transported second and

those with minor injuries
are the last to be treated and
transported.

U

Unconditional Positive Regard
Treating patients with respect
and dignity and viewing them
as worthy and capable, even
when they do not act or feel
that way.

W

Workers Compensation
Insurance to cover medical care
and compensation for employees
who are injured in the course of
performing their job.

Z

Zyban The brand name for the
antidepressant medication
Bupropion. It is prescribed for
tobacco cessation.

Zyprexa The brand name for
the atypical antipsychotic
medication Olanzapine.

Index

A